CANCER STORIES

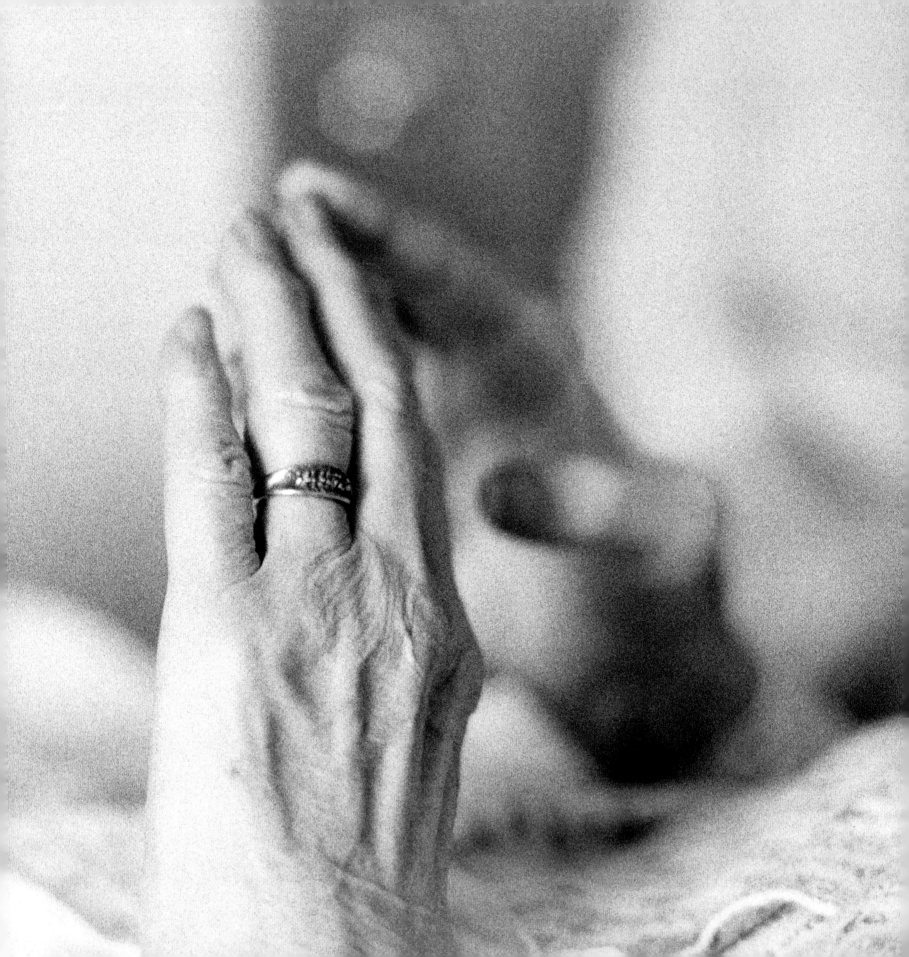

CANCER STORIES

Lessons in Love, Loss & Hope

EDITED BY JOHN TEMPLE AND JOEL BEESON

Published by WEST VIRGINIA UNIVERSITY PRESS

for THE PERLEY ISAAC REED SCHOOL OF JOURNALISM

& THE MARY BABB RANDOLPH CANCER CENTER

10 09 08 07 06 05 04   8 7 6 5 4 3 2 1

ISBN 0-937058-88-2 (alk. paper)

Library of Congress Cataloguing-in-Publication Data

Cancer stories. Lessons in love, loss & hope/ [edited] by John Temple and Joel Beeson.
x, 222 p. 120 illus. 26 cm.
1. Journalism. 2. Photojournalism 3. Interviews. 4. Journalism—Medical. 5. Quality of Life.
6. Quality of Health Care. 7. Health Behavior. 8. Cancer—Social Aspects. 9. Cancer Treatment.
10. Journalism—Educational. I. Title. II. Temple, John. III. Beeson, Joel.

IN PROCESS

Library of Congress Control Number: 2004113379

Designed by Dana Coester
Type set in 11/17 Goudy
Printed by C & C Offset Printing Co., Ltd.
Printed in China

IN HONOR AND MEMORY OF

Fred Arnold,
George Catselis &
Kathern Polen Steele

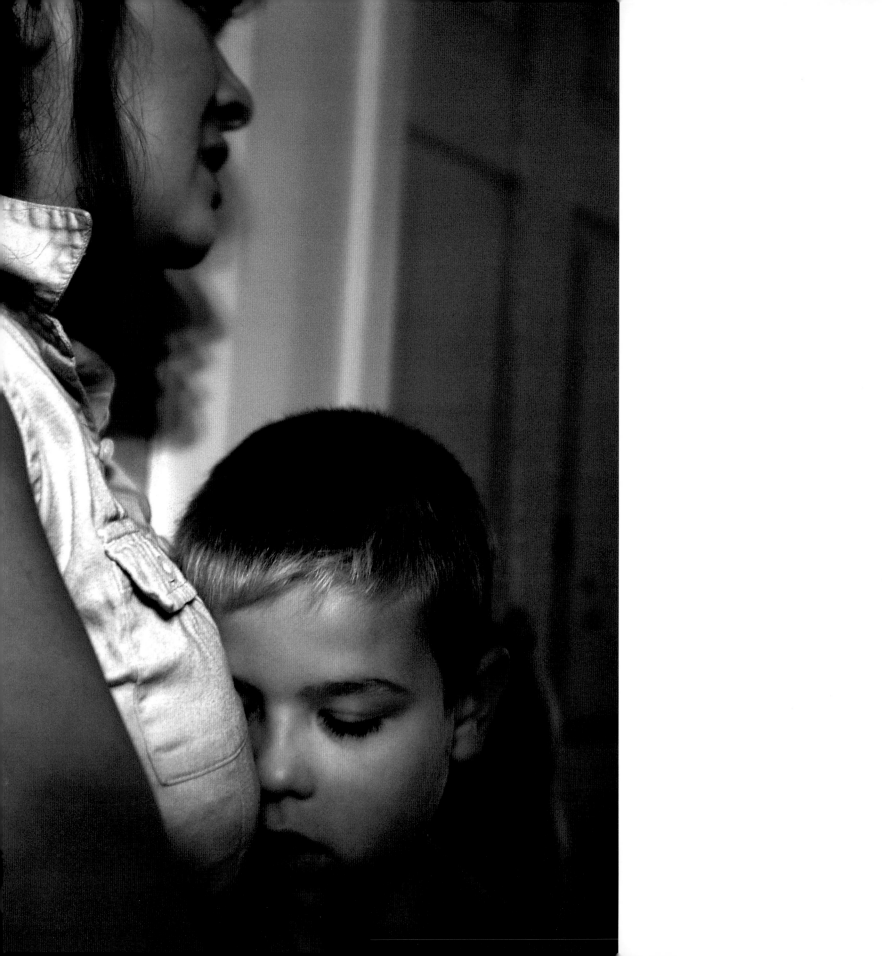

TABLE *of* CONTENTS

(opposite) "I think a woman's breasts define more than just one thing. Sexuality is one purpose, but they are also maternal. I always wanted to breast-feed my babies. I was their lifeline, their source for food. But my breasts also define me as a woman." TAMMEY MASON, BREAST CANCER SURVIVOR

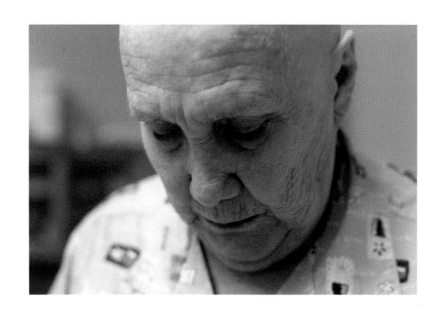

This book is purely a labor of passion and love.

In fact, I have never known a truer example of love's labor than what we, the students and faculty of the Perley Isaac Reed School of Journalism, have come to call The Cancer Project.

The Cancer Project was born from a letter sent to West Virginia University President David C. Hardesty. David Allen, a longtime supporter of the Mary Babb Randolph Cancer Center, suggested that the School of Journalism partner with the Cancer Center to create a series of stories that chronicle the lives of cancer patients from diagnosis through treatment. The stories would offer an intimate, compassionate, unflinching record of each person's struggle with cancer.

When I received the letter from President Hardesty, I loved the idea. I especially loved the suggestion that the School of Journalism students serve as the chroniclers of the patients' stories. David Allen believed that the students' vision—un-jaded, un-biased, trusting and pure—would allow the students to practice caring, precise, and honest journalism with no cynicism or strings attached.

The next step was to meet with Eddie Reed, MD, the Cancer Center director, who turned out to be another visionary who believed in David Allen's idea. He envisioned journalism students and faculty forming a unique partnership with the patients, doctors, and nurses at his Cancer

Center. And he knew that partnership would not only produce fine journalism but also produce fine public service and fine patient care.

Dr. Reed's hope, like our own, was to produce a book and a documentary film that would offer information, help, and solace to cancer patients, doctors, families, friends, West Virginians—to everyone who has been touched in any way by cancer.

Eddie Reed, David Allen, and his brother John pledged full support to the School of Journalism. Pubic relations CEO and founder of The Arnold Agency, Linda Arnold, also offered her support for the project. In return, the school offered the commitment of our faculty and the hard and good work of its students.

Together we devoted three years to telling the stories of the most courageous, compassionate, and extraordinary people we have ever met—the cancer patients—who agreed to open their hearts, their home and their lives to this project.

None of us knew what we were in for when we started. None of us knew how hard or how wonderful or how pivotal this project would become professionally and personally. What began as an idea became a lesson in partnership, in trust, in patience, and in love. The result of this extraordinary ensemble—this symphony of vision and voices—is an Emmy-winning documentary film and the following book.

But the result for all of us has been so much more than we could ever imagine. David Allen said in his initial proposal, "As with all such projects, we will learn far more than we think we will at the outset."

We have. This lesson has changed how we practice journalism, and it has changed how we practice life.

by CHRISTINE MARTIN
EXECUTIVE DIRECTOR, "THE CANCER PROJECT"

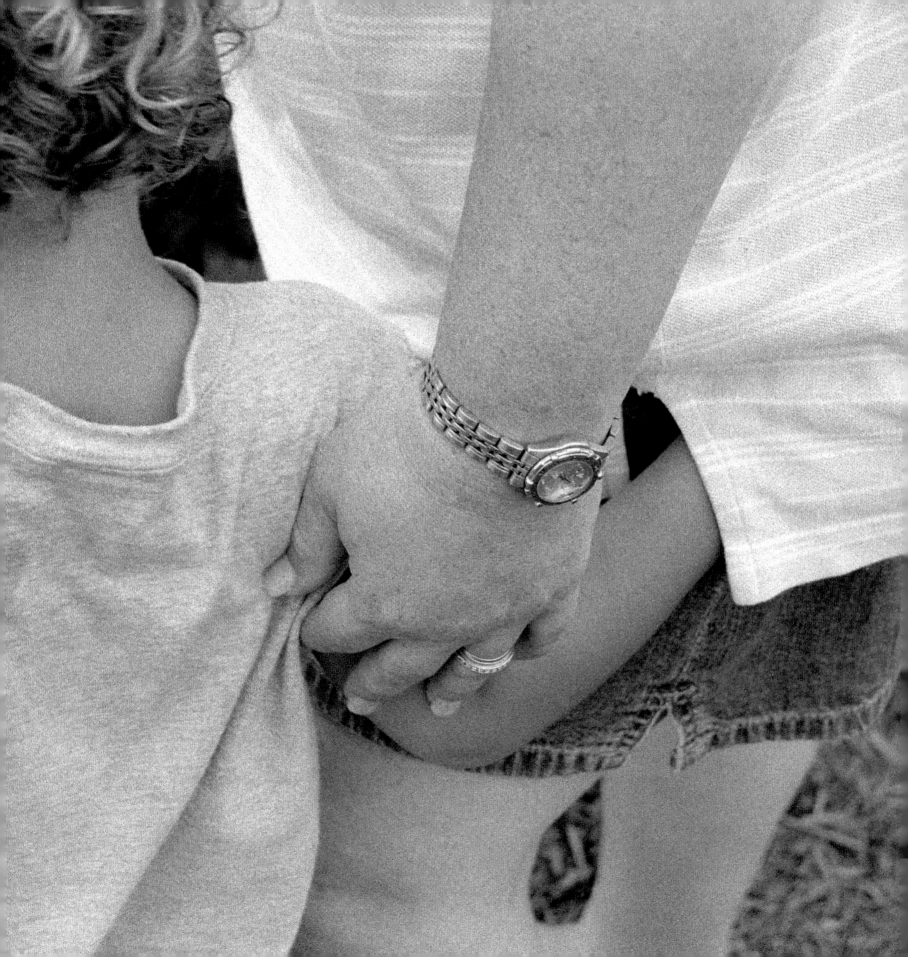

My cancer experience began with this book.

Cancer was not something I'd thought about as a senior in college. I knew I wanted to write, and the idea of immersing myself into another's life for a year set my journalistic spirit soaring. But the events to come would far exceed my simple expectations.

During the first months of the cancer project, as we called it, oncologists lectured the writers about cancer and escorted us through cold treatment rooms. Finally, I was teamed with a willing subject. I was the last to get a patient.

Dr. Jame Abraham told me that Pam Tsuhlares was a 40-something artist with an aggressive form of breast cancer. And he almost seemed protective of her, hesitant to let her fragile life be invaded by a young journalist. I didn't blame him.

I was naïve, as many of us were. I never expected such a beautiful person as Pam, nor such normalcy in a life lived with cancer.

When I first met Pam, she had already lost her hair and an inch of blonde had grown back all around her head. She had already lost her breasts and many surrounding lymph nodes. Her redheaded side-kick sister, Jody, was right beside her the whole time, no matter what.

Pam extended a warm hand and smile to me from day one. I was with her during her radiation appointments, chemotherapy, at Jody's where she'd stay while in Morgantown, at her home in Wheeling, and, at times, away from it all, just having something to eat.

Pam's gentle nature was reflected by the collection of wind chimes outside her home, her charcoal drawings, and her blue eyes, which would light up with joy or dim when she was in pain.

I remember the hardest four days, which eventually framed my chapter, the days when hope and fear were most intense—the days when Pam's prognosis teetered between remission and death. The disease had spread to her liver, and a radical surgery involving burning the tumors could give her a clean slate or induce liver failure. But Pam, Jody, Pam's husband Lambros, and her children were eager for a life without cancer.

The day she came out of the surgery was the hardest day, and something Pam and Jody could not joke off, as they usually did so well. Pam was in ICU, and pale, dried blood laced her lips from the tube down her throat. She was unable to speak except to moan.

Even though they called me "friend," and they had done all they could to welcome me in, I didn't want to hold the tape recorder anymore. I felt the burn of that experience for days. I came home that day and took a bath, just staring into space. I mourned for what she'd had to go through. Her body had been cut and sewn and poked and probed and radiated and pumped with poison, and it wasn't over yet.

Something that brought me out of that mourning was to sit down and write it out. It was my longest piece of writing to that date.

For allowing me to experience all that I did in the creation of *Cancer Stories*, I thank the participating oncologists at the Mary Babb Randolph Cancer Center. Its director, Dr. Eddie Reed, helped inspire and organize the project, along with the cooperation of a number of cancer center physicians, including Drs. Jame Abraham, Miklos Auber, Solveig Ericson, Marcel Devetten, Ankesh Nigam, John Rogers, and Andrew Soisson. They are truly gifted and dedicated to their honorable profession.

I thank the Perley Isaac Reed School of Journalism and the knowledgeable cancer project advisors: John Temple, Joel Beeson, Maryanne Reed, George Esper, Leslie Rubinkowski, and Clint Wilhelm; and the many students who worked on this project. I'd also like to extend a special thanks to Dean Christine Martin for tirelessly pursuing the vision of David Allen, a major early sponsor and initiator of the project. And many thanks to Linda Arnold, chief executive officer of The Arnold Agency, whose generous donation made this book possible.

Last but not least, I'd like to honor the true heroes, the cancer patients. This experience will continue to be etched into my heart. God bless.

by JENNIFER ROUSH

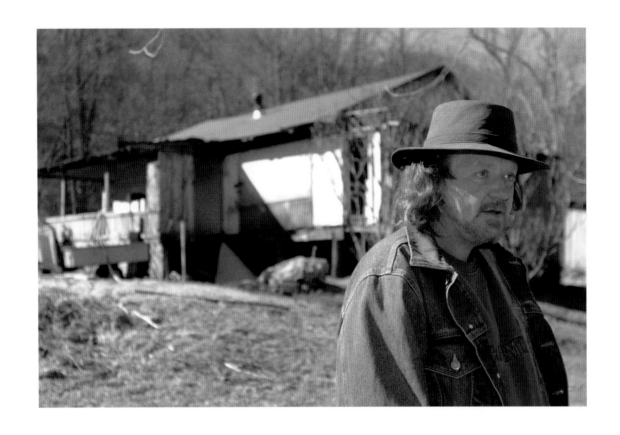

HE KEEPS GOING

text by GRANT SMITH

It's a Monday morning, May 2002, and Tim Grounds wakes early, feeling fine. As soon as he pulls himself up from the bed, though, his shoulder starts throbbing. It's a constant, dull throb, reminiscent of his surgeries. He takes a painkiller, Percocet, and goes to wake up his kids. Today is a school day, and they can't be late. He sees the kids off to school, and then gets ready for his workday. Today the job at hand is the same as every school day: drive to Morgantown, get his cancer treatment, drive back in time to be home for his kids when school lets out.

Tim hobbles into his little Metro and drives down the road a bit to pick up coffee from McDonalds or the Sheetz Quick Stop. They all know him there, almost as well as they know him at the West Virginia University Mary Babb Randolph Cancer Center in Morgantown, today's destination.

Tim drives down the strip past the Potomac Valley Hospital, past West Virginia University Potomac State, past homes and gas stations, and makes his way to Route 220.

Timothy Grounds is a fighter, and in 2001 he began the fight of his life. Diagnosed with stage III melanoma days after Christmas, Tim began his struggle not only with his cancer, but with the rest of his life. In the years since his diagnosis, Tim has seen divorce. He has seen child custody battles and financial hardships. A.J., Tim's son, reflects on his father's life, "He's all beat up, but he keeps going."

photographs by MELISSA NETHKEN

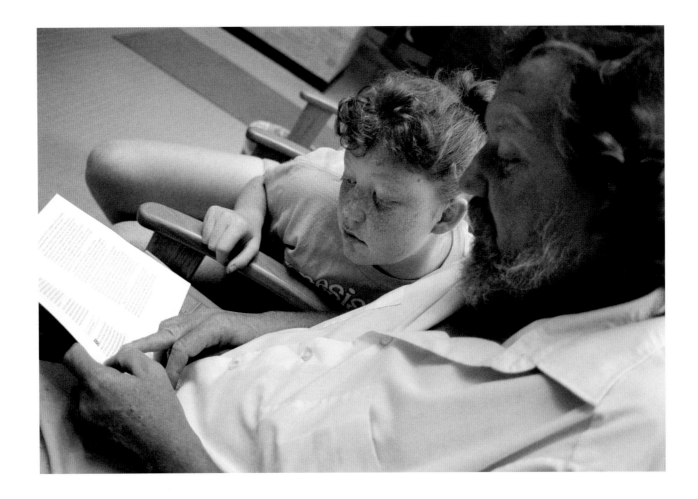

While waiting for an interferon treatment at the Mary Babb Randolph Cancer Center, Tim shares a brochure with his daughter, Nikki, describing types of people who may be at risk for melanoma. Nikki is like her father in many ways—always quick to make a joke and friendly to everyone around her. Nikki has also inherited Tim's pale skin and red hair, features that prompt Tim to warn her about being safe in the sun.

The road isn't bad, not nearly as winding as the road to Webster Springs. Not nearly as long, either. He'll stay on this road for another 45 minutes until he hits the interstate, where he'll drive another 45 minutes to Morgantown. It's a three hour, 170-mile round-trip that Tim makes five days a week.

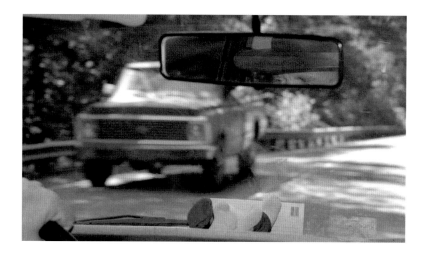

In summer 2001, six months before he found out about the melanoma, Tim was a blue-collar man who worked too hard and too often to be with his family as much as anyone would have liked. He is a man who spent long hours in the sawmill and mowed lawns at night to support his family. Tim is no stranger to hard work and no man to complain. But by late fall, he and his wife Tammy had separated, leaving him alone in Webster Springs to take care of A.J., 14, and Nikki, 12.

But his story goes back further than that.

When Tim was a kid, the two sets of nerves in his neck that control each hand merged together, and ever since, what one hand does, the other mimics. On Parris Island with the Marines, he did what they told him because he had to. But when they told him to climb down a 30-foot rope, he told them, "Sorry, Sir, I cannot do that."

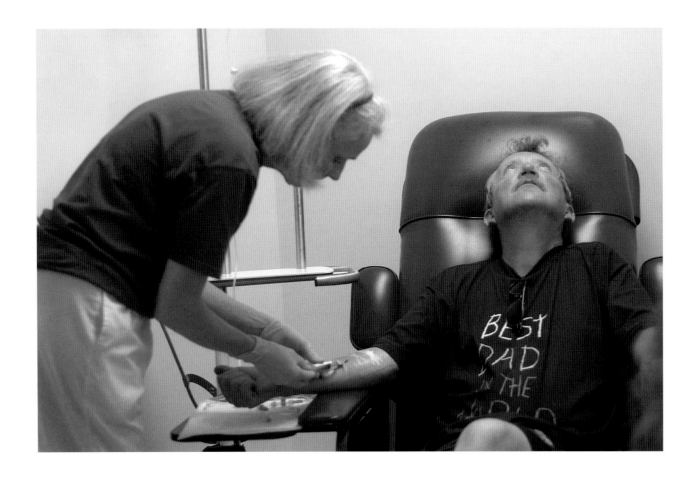

In May 2002, Tim underwent chemotherapy treatments. The initial site of the cancer was removed, and now Tim must travel from Keyser to Morgantown several times a week for his treatments. For Tim, the worst part isn't until he gets home. Unwilling to rest as he is advised to do, Tim finds himself sick more often than not, sometimes ending up in the local hospital for help with pain and nausea.

Photo by Jason DeProspero

But he did it anyway. He tried to climb down that rope, and when one hand opened up to move down the rope, the other opened up, too, and Tim fell. He was pretty badly hurt, but he mended.

Tim always fought to do whatever was required of him, and he did it till it broke him.

———

Tim looks forward to the day when his treatment in Morgantown is over, when he'll start getting shots of a lower dosage three times a week at the hospital in Keyser. There, it's less than a two-minute drive from his trailer to the hospital. A nurse explained to Tim that the lower doses of interferon he'll get from the shots keep "kicking the body" to boost its ability to fight the cancer.

But for the time being, Tim continues to drive to the Mary Babb Randolph Cancer Center in Morgantown for his treatment five days a week, because he can't get it in Keyser. When he gets to the Cancer Center, if it's a Monday, like today, they'll take him back to an open area and weigh him, take his blood pressure, and then take blood samples to test if his white blood cell count is good enough to get the treatment this week. If it's the first Monday of the month, they do a bunch of tests, the "full scan," Tim says. But today is the third week of the month, so he only gets one test. After nurses load a couple tubes with his blood, they take him back to an open cubicle-like room where he'll wait for the test results, and then he'll wait for them to hook him up to the drip machine. Today though, they are busy. He sits in a chair and waits for the nurses to get to him.

"Can you use a cell phone in here?" he asks nobody in particular.

A nurse tells him to go ahead, but not to talk very long. He calls his bank back in Webster County, and tells the person on the other end that he's got a problem with his account. There's a problem with his house payment, and someone applied a payment to his account that should have been applied to his ex-wife's.

The person on the other line doesn't seem to understand and puts him on hold. Tim smacks his forehead and looks around, disgusted. He greets the person still slightly annoyed.

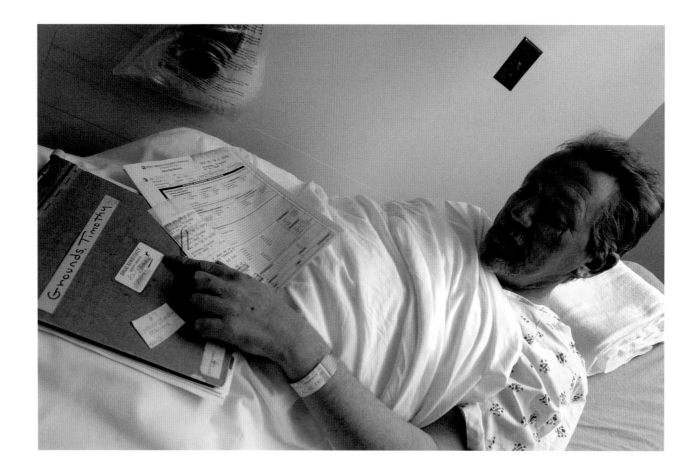

Tim's medical treatments not only bring a physical burden but also a financial one. No longer able to work due to his illness, Tim relies solely on Social Security as his main income, which does not go far. His frequent trips to Morgantown put a large dent in the money he has left over after paying his monthly bills. The hospital's social worker assists Tim frequently with seeking additional funding. For Tim, this means lots of paperwork and waiting to get any results.

Photo by Brian Persinger

"… it only makes sense that if she's $80 behind and I'm $80 ahead that somebody put it in the wrong account," he says into the phone.

Tim's had money troubles. He can't work, and when he and his wife split up and he got cancer, he had nothing saved up. He makes approximately $1,200 a month from Social Security, but by the time he pays bills, he's only got about $500 left. He lives paycheck to pay-

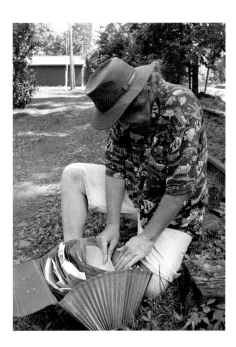

check and has a rough time making ends meet. The social services department at the Cancer Center has helped him apply for different types of funding.

Before he has his blood drawn, the nurse asks him, as she does every day, if he took his Tylenol before he came.

His reply is always the same: "Yes, ma'am. I'm a good boy."

Today, like most days, the test results came back OK. His treatment arrives in a clear bag, runs through a tube into a machine that controls the rate of flow and then into a valve in his forearm. The valve connects to a thin tube, or pick-line, that runs up his arm into his chest, within an inch of his heart. They take blood samples from this tube, too. After the nurses take the blood, they flush the tube with saline, saltwater, to prevent blood clots or buildup. He hates the saltwater and somehow tastes it almost immediately. He grimaces.

"That's nasty!" Tim says, as he scrunches his face in disgust.

They will flush the pick-line with saline again after the bag is empty.

He looks at the bag of interferon that's dripping through the tube into his arm now, slightly concerned and annoyed. It's cloudy white.

"The pamphlet thing I got said it was supposed to be clear," Tim mumbles.

Early in Tim's treatment, he became dizzy and nauseous, vomiting regularly, and ended up in the hospital for a few days. Normally, the nurses just turn on one bag of interferon, but this time, Tim says, they had a bag of that dreaded saline running.

"I thought that was it for me," Tim recalls. "I didn't think I was coming back."

Tim had quite a scare from his treatment. Patients receiving interferon aren't supposed to be in the sun very much; doing so can lower their white blood cell or potassium count. Tim says he didn't know that. Whether he forgot or wasn't informed, those levels dropped, and he periodically "went blind." As he described it, his field of vision got smaller and smaller, until all he saw was black. This could be dangerous if, for instance, he were driving. He got a computerized axial tomography (CAT) scan of his brain to check and see if anything abnormal was going on up there, but they told Tim it was probably his medicine. Fortunately it was the interferon and the sun exposure. Miklos Auber, MD, Tim's oncologist in Morgantown, reduced his dosage.

Tim was 41 years old when he was diagnosed with malignant melanoma skin cancer. Not all skin cancers are melanomas, which develop from the skin cells called melanocytes that produce the skin pigment melanin. Melanoma is generally more serious than other skin cancers, but it is almost always curable if caught early, although it can easily spread to other parts of the body. Dr. Auber says Tim's melanoma was about 10 millimeters thick before it was caught. The cancer had spread to the lymph nodes in what is known as stage III melanoma.

Melanoma is classified into four stages. The Melanoma Patients' Information Page (http://www.mpip.org) explains stage I melanoma as a skin cancer where the tumor is only 1.5 millimeters deep, existing only in the outer skin layer or the upper part of the inner layer of skin. Stage II melanoma spreads a little deeper, up to 4 millimeters, but it hasn't spread to other body tissues. Stage III melanoma is like Tim's cancer. In fourth stage melanoma, the cancer has spread into the body's organs, in addition to the lymph nodes.

Tim noticed a mole-like spot behind his left shoulder in fall 2001. After only four months, it became easily irritated and looked as though it would bleed if you scratched it the least little bit. It even became difficult to sleep on.

In 2002 alone, according to American Cancer Society statistics, an estimated 53,600 people were diagnosed with melanoma in the United States; approximately 7,400 people died. That accounts for approximately 10 percent of new cancer cases and approximately 1.5 percent of cancer deaths in 2002. The statistical odds of surviving seem pretty good, but Tim's cancer is fairly developed, which reduces his overall chances of staying cancer free.

The treatment Tim will receive is common for stage III melanoma. Most patients have surgery to remove the skin melanoma, and if the lymph nodes in the area of the melanoma feel hard or abnormally large, they are cut out and evaluated for cancer cells. After all cancer cells have been removed, interferon alpha is administered to boost the immune system and to keep the cancer from coming back.

Interferon is a "biologic response modifier" used to stimulate the immune system and boost the body's ability to fight the disease by increasing the number of tumor-killing cells, according to MerckSource, an online Merck Manual resource. Interferon can also directly attack and destroy cancerous tumors.

Tim has undergone four surgeries so far. The first surgery was to remove the melanoma spot on his shoulder, and it wasn't really a success. Tim says the edges of the removed piece weren't clean, meaning they contained spots of cancer. The edges from a successful surgery should be normal tissue with no cancer, meaning the surgeon was able to go around it and cut it all out.

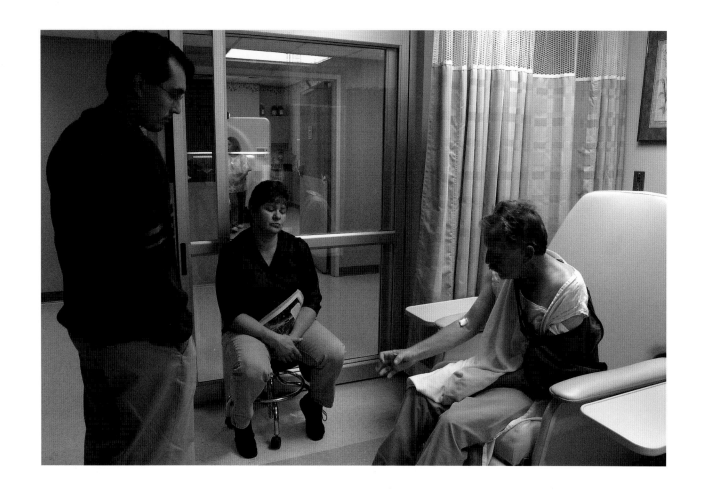

The left side of Tim's body has suffered greatly. Waiting for a CAT scan with his friend Cindy, Tim wears a sling to support his left arm. Tim has had multiple surgeries to remove the cancer from his shoulder. His lymph nodes have been removed from under his left arm and he has fallen twice on the same side, fracturing his collarbone.

Photo by Karina Gomes Dick

So Tim had a second surgery in Morgantown to remove the rest of the melanoma. This one was successful: the edges were clean. The melanoma was deep though, so he had another surgery to check for cancer in the closest lymph nodes to the melanoma, the ones in his left armpit. The doctor found a little bit of cancer and cut into him again to see if there was any more, but he found only inflammation.

——

Tim's best friend Cindy has known him since junior high. She categorizes her friendship with Tim as deep, one that you don't come by too many times, one that she truly cherishes. Cindy and Tim can talk about anything. Cindy says he's like the brother she never had or like a girlfriend she can confide in that just happens to be a guy.

Cindy will tell you that Tim is real fighter, and he's hardheaded, too.

He fought hard, fought to get his son A.J. from his mother, Tim's first wife, and he fought to provide for his family. He worked hard.

Tim worked for a time in Huttonsville as a deputy sheriff. He was also a jailer and a dispatcher for the State Police in Webster Springs. Cindy used to work in the State Police headquarters with Tim, and she recalls seeing him work the radio and two phones, all at the same time. If an officer was out for a while and hadn't checked in, Tim would radio around and track him down. She says he was the best dispatcher they had ever seen, but eventually Tim's hardheadedness got in the way. He butted heads with the recently elected sheriff, and he was fired.

Tim was clearing brush after a flood in Webster Springs a couple years ago, and a log he was sawing twisted around and smashed his knee against a rock, breaking his kneecap and tearing cartilage.

He was set to undergo knee replacement surgery until he learned that he had cancer.

"The doctor said there ain't no use to fix it until I find out if I'm gonna live long enough to use it," Tim says.

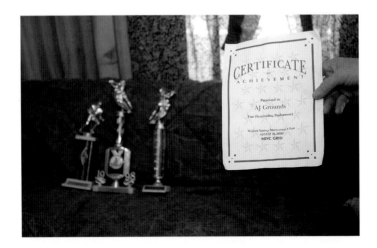

To this day, Tim's kneecap does not line up straight with his leg. It hasn't bothered him lately though, since he's taking so many painkillers.

Cindy talks about Tim, remembering the good times, and thinking about the future. She talks about how reliable Tim is, his commitment to his friends. She talks about how he'll be there for his friends, helping them out, doing what they need. She talks about how, when things take a turn for the worse, Tim takes it in stride. But she also talks about how Tim can't help his friends out any more, and how he needs them more now than they need him.

"Tim's been there," Cindy says, "He's always been there …"

She speaks with sadness, tears welling up in her eyes. She speaks with sadness because Tim may not be there much longer.

Tim is not the only one affected by his illness. His children, who reside with him, also have a hard time dealing with it. "The kids are not taking it too good. It's hard on 'em, real hard on 'em." However, even in their hard times, Tim is quick to show visitors their trophies and awards and to point out their accomplishments.

It is no surprise what Tim did when he was told he might die in six months. He talked to his friend. Tim drove up to Cindy's home in Keyser and stayed the night.

"Cindy, she was real upset and cried a lot," Tim recalls.

Cindy's husband called a doctor friend of his and had him explain the biopsy results, while Tim and Cindy sat in the kitchen for a while, drinking coffee before moving to the living room. Cindy's teenage daughter Stephanie says Tim is a person who really holds onto memories, and Cindy says he's brought so many memories back to her. Since he started his treatment though, he's been uncharacteristically forgetful. But Tim still remembers how they looked at old pictures and talked about old times that night. About times back in Webster Springs, when he was a dispatcher, about good times before he and his wife split up and before he got cancer. As he talks about those days, he gets out an old cookie tin filled with pictures and starts thumbing through them.

He flips through pictures of his brothers and sisters, his parents, A.J., Nikki; pictures of holidays and co-workers; pictures of the kids playing, making goofy faces; pictures of his ex-wife Tammy's daughter Ashley; and pictures of Tammy with the kids.

He looks sad. Today would have been their 15th anniversary. Then he laughs and says that he called her up that morning and wished her a happy anniversary.

"She didn't say nothin'. She hung up."

He laughs again.

Tim's life changed forever when she left him. So did A.J.'s and Nikki's.

"The kids are not taking it too good," Tim says. "It's hard on 'em, real hard on 'em."

He drove back to Webster the day after his visit to Keyser and ran into a bit of car trouble. He topped a hill, and he just "burnt the clutch plumb out of it." Tim loves his vehicles, but they seem to give him a lot of trouble.

He bought a Geo Metro a few months ago for $400 and souped it up. It's not souped up engine-wise, but it looks pretty sharp. He put a FEAR THIS sticker on the top of the windshield, and he stuck a propeller below the rear bumper and a pretty sharp-looking fake air-intake in the center of the hood. Cleaned the engine up quite a bit, too, and painted the block

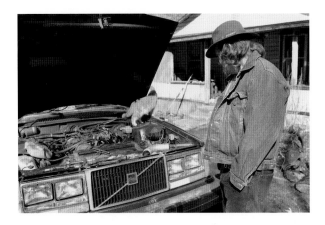

Chevy orange. With all the driving to his appointments in Morgantown and trips to Webster Springs, Tim has put 27,000 miles on his Geo in only six or seven months.

Right before school let out in 2002, he bought an old Dodge truck to take his kids camping. He since traded that truck to his brother for an old Ford Metro. He doesn't drive it around that often because it burns oil and doesn't get very good gas mileage.

Tim likes to put the pedal down, and he's had a few accidents in that Metro. He was coming down the mountain near Webster Springs, hit a slick spot in the road and spun out into the guardrail. The Metro took a beating that day, and he'll wreck again in a few weeks. Tim won't be able to stop in time when a woman pulls her car into his lane and stops. Both headlights are slightly bashed in; the propeller and one tailpipe are both missing. The other tailpipe is bent sideways. The little car still runs pretty well, though.

AJ is generally not very vocal about his dad but adamantly proclaims how Tim is just like his cars. "He's all beat up," he says, "but he keeps going."

Tim's just like his dad, too, he says. The years have worn on the elder Grounds, too. He walks with an obvious limp, and one eyebrow droops so low you wonder if that eye does him any good at all. He's quick to make a joke and even quicker to dig up a batch of potatoes for a guest to take home. He's wrecked his four-wheeler a few times but still likes to fishtail it in the gravel at high speeds.

Tim's dad was injured in a mine accident, and Tim says most of the bones in his body were broken, including his legs and hips. He says his dad just learned to walk again "one step at a time," as if there were any other way, as if there were never any doubt about him walking again.

Tim will follow his dad's example and just fight cancer one step at a time.

———

Pictures of Tim a few years ago show him as a thin man, always smiling. He isn't very tall, but he's healthy looking, strong and happy. Now at 43, Tim looks worn down.

Unshaven more often than not, his mustachioed face is creased, his eyes are tired, and his smile is slower to take shape. Tim grew up without a shirt on, and it shows in the permanent sunburned redness on his chest. The years of hard work show too. They show in the roughness of his hands from changing big rig tires for years, first at a truck stop, and later, at his own business in a gravel lot across the river from his parents' and brother's homes. His fingernails are ridged, and the backs of his hands scarred and aged. His arms are dark and freckled.

More than anything, though, the months with cancer show.

Tim's lost weight, and he's less muscular than he used to be. His weight fluctuates from 143 pounds to 157 pounds in a week. He breaks into a sweat easily doing simple tasks like the laundry, and occasionally, when Tim works himself too hard, he'll get hot or dizzy and black out. He's fallen on his shoulder at least twice, once onto the unforgiving asphalt, onto the same shoulder where he had surgery to remove the melanoma. And he had his lymph nodes removed under that same shoulder. The doctor says he's got a hairline fracture in his collarbone, and all the tissues are inflamed and swollen. He's taking an anti-inflammatory medicine that occasionally turns his normally bloodshot eyes a jaundiced yellow.

———

Tim's hometown, Webster Springs, is a small coal mining and lumber town that fits snug between two mountains with a river running down the middle. The road to Webster is long and narrow and winds up and down the mountains. If you're not careful at night, you'll hit a deer crossing the road.

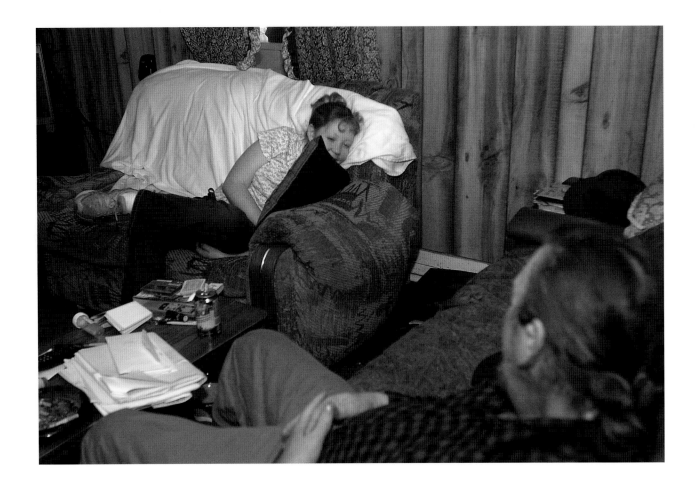

Amid the struggle in Tim's life, there is always laughter. "You gotta keep a sense of humor," he says, "If you don't, it'll kill you." Both of his children are an endless source of laughter for Tim. Nikki is completely open with her father, sharing stories about her latest crush while she giggles behind a pillow she made that same day.

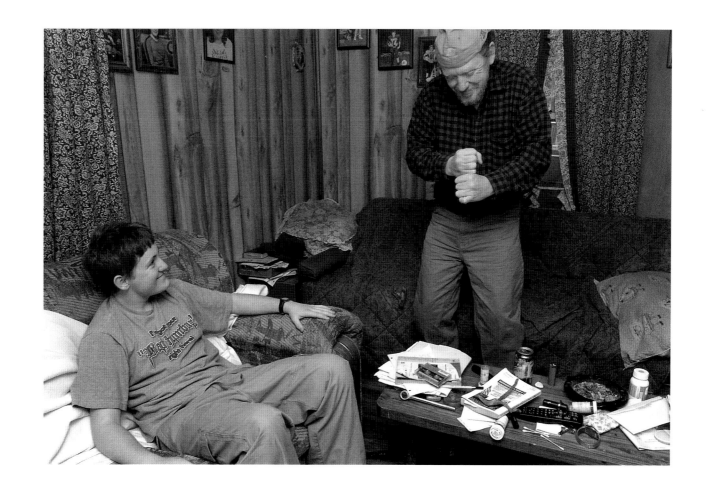

A.J. is also a source of humor in the house. He and his father feed off one another's jokes. While Tim dances around, A.J. tries to guess who Tim is impersonating.

There's not much out there, though, other than the woods and the Elk River.

Tim has lived here all his life.

Cindy will tell you it's a wonderful hometown, but it doesn't offer much for kids to do. The nearest McDonalds or hospital is 45 minutes away. No bowling alleys or indoor recreation, just the great outdoors. Tim and his kids live right on the Elk, across from the main road, down-river from his parents and sister's houses.

It's a sparsely populated area located in a county with approximately 10,000 people, according to a 1990 state census, and Cindy says everyone kind of sticks together, afraid to move on. She did move on, though, up north to Keyser, her husband's hometown. Tim moved to Keyser, too, finally, after he learned he had cancer. He wanted to be closer to Cindy and to his treatment in Morgantown.

"They told me to move up here, and I said I'd think about it," Tim explains. "Next month I did move up here."

Tim, A.J., and Nikki moved into a small, narrow trailer in Keyser, a couple blocks from Cindy's house, near the Sheetz Quick Stop and the hospital. The screen in the door is broken, and flies pass freely through. They have an air conditioner but can't run much else in the house at the same time or the circuit breaker kicks the power off. It's not too comfortable, but it's convenient.

———

For God so loved the world that he gave his only Son, so that everyone who believes in him may not die but have eternal life. — JOHN 3:16

Tim is getting ready to go down to Webster Springs for a few days and says he's looking forward to Sunday school. Since Tim and his kids moved up to Keyser, they haven't gone to church, unless they happen to be in Webster on a Sunday. Cindy thinks that fact really bothers him. Tim says he just hasn't found a church in Keyser like the one back home in Webster.

"I kinda been letting the Lord down … " he admits.

Tammy and the kids went to church long before he ever did, but toward the beginning of

November 2001, right before Tammy left him and less than two months before he learned he had cancer, Tim finally started going to church.

"I read the whole Bible," Tim says. "Lot of good stuff in the Bible."

About that time, Tim began to take a hard look at his drinking.

"Tim drank a lot, he really did," Cindy says. "Got to the point he was drinking almost all the time."

Cindy said he always had a beer in his hand when he was mowing grass or otherwise. Tim admits he drank "his share … and somebody else's."

Sudden Infant Death Syndrome, commonly known as SIDS, or "crib death," claimed Tim and Tammy's first baby girl when she was three months old.

After Tammy and Tim's first baby died, Cindy says he started drinking more, using drinking as a crutch.

"If he wasn't an alcoholic, he was on his way to becoming one," Cindy explains.

"Hardest thing is burying one of your own children, even harder than this [cancer]," he says.

Eventually, Tim told Tammy he would quit drinking, and that's exactly what he did.

"He went out on the railroad tracks and asked God to take it away, and he was saved," Cindy says. "He's got a good rapport with God and accepted God into his life."

Tim's faith has played no small role in his fight with cancer. He'll tell you that he "just felt it was time" to quit drinking and start going to church, and it sure seems like it was just in time. He doesn't know if he could have even accepted the reality of his cancer if not for his faith in the Lord. He attributes most of his survival so far to God.

"Faith in the Lord has gotten me this far," Tim says. "He could've taken me right on out of this life, but he didn't."

Sometimes, the kids take care of Tim. They help around the house, picking up, and they watch out for their dad when he gets sick. Tim recalls a day he was napping when Nikki went down to the store to pick up a cake mix to surprise him.

But kids being kids, they probably don't help as much as they should.

"We've all had a talk with them about helping Tim around the house," Cindy says. "I think they are going through a lot too with what their dad is going through."

He's thankful, though, for all he's got.

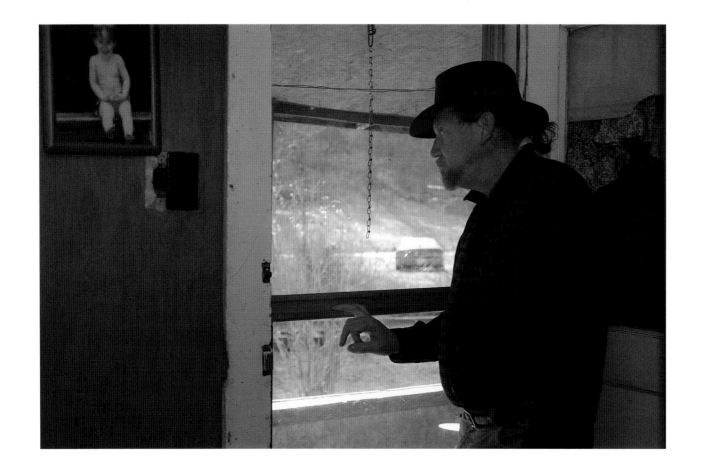

Tim has known hard work his whole life. Now most days he sits at home, watching the morning television line-up, old shows like Gunsmoke and The Waltons. He passes the time with solitaire, a game he claims never to have lost, and talks with the neighbors. The highlight of the day is when his kids come home on the school bus.

Having gone to the Cancer Center for a while, Tim has seen the pain other people bear.

"I guess most of them there aren't doing as good as I am," he says.

Cindy thinks he's doing pretty well, considering everything he's been going through.

"I think Tim deals with all of this easier than I would … I think he deals with it on a basis that he has to because of his children. He deals with it a whole lot better than I ever expected."

Tim hasn't been doing everything right though. Things have changed since he began getting his shots in Keyser.

—————

Tim is done with his five-day-a-week interferon treatment, and the next step will be high doses of interferon intravenously, to help the body fight the growth of his cancer.

Tim wakes up to get his kids ready for school. The shoulder still hurts when he gets out of bed, mostly now because of his fractured collarbone, and the shoulder tissue is still inflamed and tender. He's fallen on it twice now and refuses to wear his arm in a sling. Every now and then, a stitch from inside his body, left over from the lymph node removal surgery, will come undone and slowly work its way to the surface. Tim can feel it happen. His side gets sore, and often gets infected and full of pus. If he pushes against the wound, little caterpillars of white pus ooze out either end of the scar.

He drives up to Cindy's for morning coffee every day. Today is no different. He'll sit and talk with Cindy and her husband for an hour or so, and then he'll head back home. If it's a Monday, Wednesday or Friday, he heads down to the hospital for his shot.

On Mondays, the nurse takes blood samples to see if he's fine for the treatment, just like Mondays in Morgantown.

As soon as the results come back, Tim gets a shot in the arm and he's done.

He's got so much free time he just doesn't know what to do with himself. He has been sick a heck of a lot more since he started getting his shots in Keyser than when he had to drive three hours everyday to Morgantown and back. It's as if he felt like he was doing something productive when he drove to Morgantown five days a week.

"I didn't slow down like they told me," Tim says. "Not being able to do something, I feel like an invalid."

"Always worked all my life … hard not to be doing anything … just so aggravated with nothin'," he trails on. "It's hard to go from being real busy all day to not able to do nothin'."

Getting cancer has actually led Tim to spend more time with his kids, but Cindy's afraid that if he doesn't start taking better care of himself and start taking it easy, he may not be around much longer to spend time with them.

Tim will have a couple of days when he feels good, and he'll go out and do something and be totally wiped out for days, or, on some occasions, end up back in the hospital.

One time he blacktopped Cindy's driveway. That night Tim was so sick and delirious he doesn't even remember going to the hospital or coming back. He remembers being hot and sweaty, then cold, and then hot again. He remembers how nauseous he was and that it felt like his feet were on fire. He doesn't even remember telling A.J. and Nikki that he loves them, and that he is dying.

———

It was no surprise that Tim ran to Cindy when he was handed his death sentence. But it is a surprise that he picked out a casket. He began making monthly payments, using his meager Social Security check to pay for it. Was Tim afraid he couldn't do what was required of him? Maybe.

Realistically, Tim may've just figured that was what was required of him this time, to make sure nobody was put out by his death any more than they had to be.

"He's scared of dying … not so much of dying, he's right with God, but scared to leave his kids and family," Cindy says.

"I gotta stick around at least to see them grow up," Tim says.

———

Tim sits on the examination table in the Cancer Center, talking to Dr. Auber, waiting for a dermatologist to check his skin.

They talk for a while about how he's doing, and the doctor re-prescribes a couple of meds for Tim: painkillers and something else for nausea. Dr. Auber tells him he should be drinking a lot of fluids to keep hydrated, and he tells Tim that may be part of the reason he gets sick so often working around the house.

As Dr. Auber gets ready to leave, Tim stops him and asks how likely it is that the cancer will return, that he won't survive this.

Relative to other cancers, not many people die from melanoma. Nonetheless, Dr. Auber says the chances of it coming back are much greater than the chances of it not coming back, especially if Tim doesn't make some lifestyle changes, like quitting smoking.

———

Tim's heart didn't feel right during one visit back to Webster, and his family took him down to the hospital in Summersville. The doctor thought his heart was out of sync and gave him electric shock therapy to put it back in rhythm.

But just a few days later, while in Morgantown for his interferon shot, Tim was complaining about his heart being out of rhythm again. Another six months were up, and he'd have to meet the $3,600 deductible again before he could get the shots in Keyser. Fortunately, or unfortunately, depending on how you look it, Tim's doctor kept him in the hospital for cardiology tests. During those couple days in the hospital he met his deductible, but he received more bad news. His heart wasn't out of rhythm; it had a hole in it.

After that Dr. Auber took him off his "maintenance" shots. Since then, Tim says he's having the same symptoms as a year ago, when he got the original biopsy. A new mole has grown back near the original melanoma. In only three weeks, it's grown to the size of a penny.

"Like it's starting all over again, watching it grow back," Tim says.

"Only, this time, with my immune system as it is …" he trails off.

A month later, Tim heads down to Morgantown for what he hopes will be his final surgery.

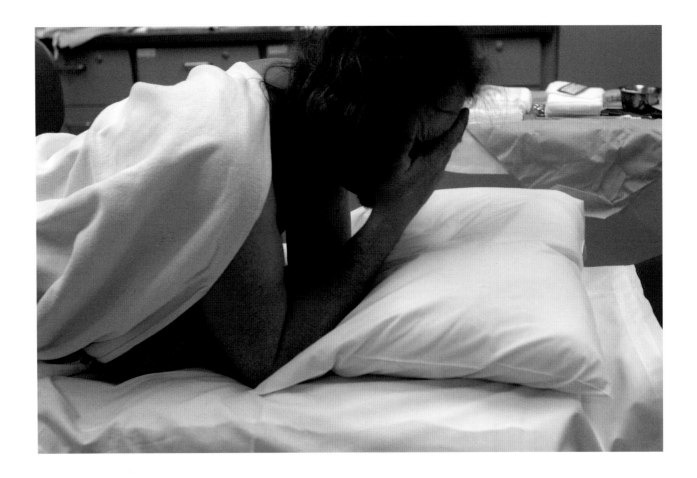

It is February 2004. A new spot has been found on Tim's neck. He discovered the spot in December, but tried to out-wit his illness by waiting until January to have it checked out. "Two times they've told me that I have cancer the day after Christmas. I figured if I waited until January it would be better news." For Tim the worst part is the numbing, a series of shots injected into his neck. It takes almost twice as long to numb the area than to perform the actual surgery.

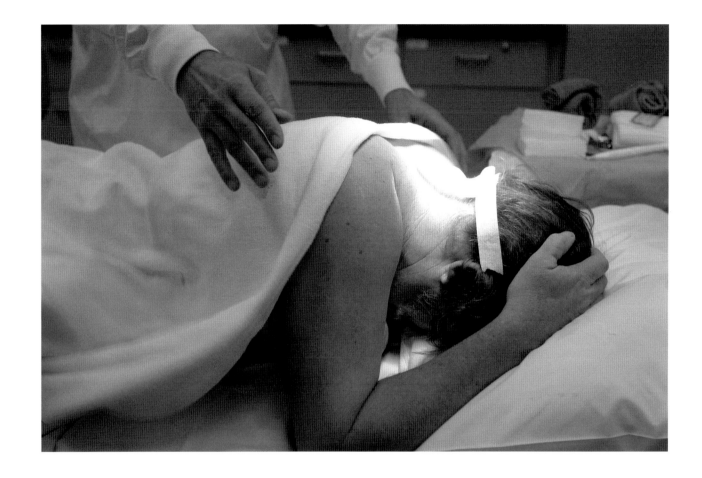

Tim's body is a battleground with scars that mark each of his triumphs. Today's surgery is outpatient, and while the spot they remove is large, the doctors see no reason for him to undergo chemotherapy or interferon treatments. They do, however, talk to him about staying out of the sun and about taking care of himself. When his surgery is finished, he gets a pat on the back and they send him back home.

Tim and the kids are sitting in the waiting room, and Tim seems tense. Nikki and A.J. have been acting up, and he's chastised them. Nikki is crying, and A.J. wanders off. It's not a good morning.

Finally, the Webster Springs clan arrives. Tim relaxes a little bit.

The goal of the surgery is to remove all the skin surrounding the reccurring cancer, to simply remove a huge chunk of flesh to test for cancer and to try to prevent any more recurrences. Dr. Auber says Tim was lucky that the new cancer spot was so close to the original spot, meaning the cancer didn't spread very far.

The surgery is successful. Doctors remove a piece of flesh approximately 14 centimeters long and 8 centimeters wide at the widest point. Skin from his thigh is grafted onto his shoulder; the hole is so big it can't just be sewn shut.

His family drives Tim and the kids back to Keyser. Now it's recovery time.

A few weeks later Tim is back at the doctor. Dr. Auber takes a look at the wound. All looks well. Dr. Auber suggests it's about time to start back on the interferon shots, once his body has healed from the surgery. Body scans and other tests don't pick up any new signs of cancer, and the cardiologist gives his approval to resume the treatment.

Tim has 20 weeks of the shots left, every Monday, Wednesday and Friday. There's a problem with his finances though, and he'll need to see the social services folks at the Cancer Center again.

After a year of ups and downs, he's back to square one. His outlook is pretty good, though. For now, he's OK.

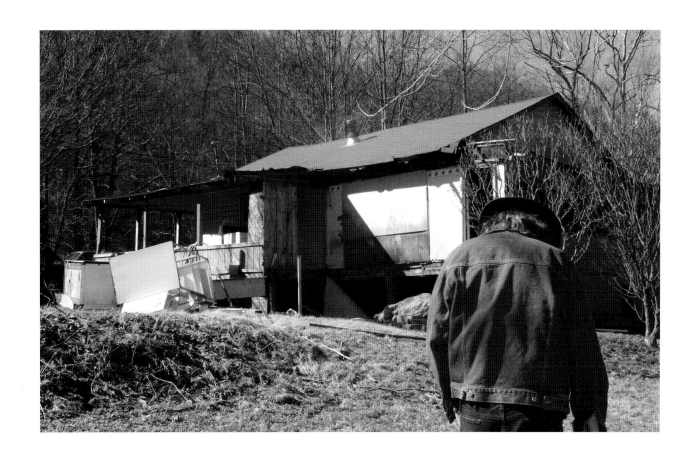

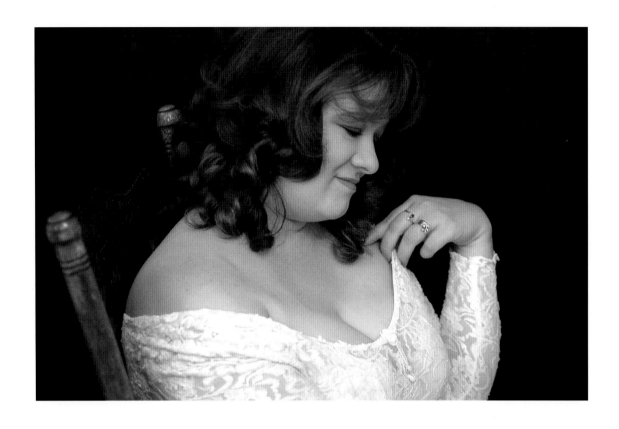

RECONSTRUCTION

text by IVY SMITH

With the push of a button, the thick wooden doors swing open. Two nurses wheel Tammey Mason's hospital bed to the first operating room. The room's pale peach walls add just enough brightness to make the transition from the dull white hallways noticeable. The sound of clanging metal fills the room as the scrub nurse organizes dozens of surgical tools on a long metal table.

After nurses help Tammey onto the operating table, the resident anesthesiologist begins hooking her to machines that will continuously read her vitals during the surgery. The steady beat of her heart is electronically reproduced in the key of C, creating a perfect cadence with the clanging metal echoing through the room as she is strapped to the operating table, and her memory begins to fade.

For the last year and half, Tammey has been piecing herself back together, and this nipple reconstruction surgery is just one more step. Though she strives for normalcy, her life has

---

Tammey Mason was diagnosed with stage I, II and III breast cancer in 2001. Within four days of her diagnosis, Tammey had a mastectomy, eight lymph nodes removed and reconstructive surgery.

photographs by LINGBING HANG

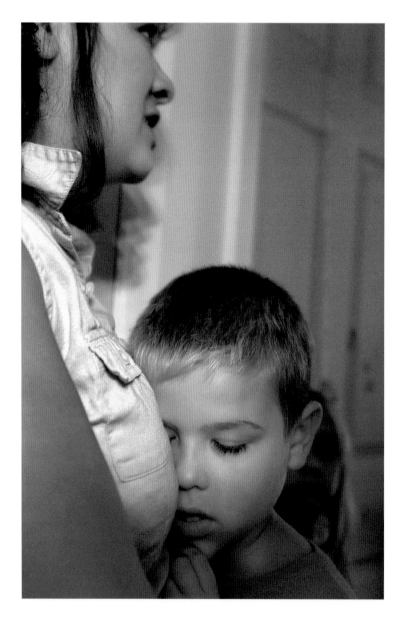

"I think a woman's breasts define more than just one thing. Sexuality is one purpose, but they are also maternal. I always wanted to breast feed my babies. I was their lifeline, their source for food. But my breasts also define me as a woman." Tammey with her son Matthew, age nine.

changed. Dark brunette hair grew in after chemotherapy, replacing her light brown locks. She gained weight fighting the disease. She lost, and then regained, her breasts. Tammey is different. She is not just a woman, but a woman who has survived breast cancer.

———

It began June 6, 2001, when 36-year-old Tammey drove to Clarksburg from her home in Salem for a routine mammogram. Doctors recommend that women begin having yearly mammograms at 40. But when Tammey, of Salem, W.Va., was pregnant with her daughter Marie four years ago, doctors found a lump on her left breast, a benign cyst, which they removed. But the lump and fibrocystic breast disease—a condition, according to *The Women's Health Companion*, found in 30 percent of women where non-cancerous lumps are present within the breast tissue—brought Tammey back for a mammogram each year.

This time Tammey's mammogram looked different. The scan of her right breast resembled a photo of stars in a night sky. The stars were clustered in three spots that looked to Tammey like galaxies.

The day of her diagnosis, Tammey went to work at Verizon Communications, where she spends hours on the phone assisting customers with telephone service problems. As she left that morning, her coworkers told her they'd see her soon.

"If it's good, you'll see me in an hour; if it's bad, you won't," she told them.

"We'll see you in an hour," they replied.

The coworkers were wrong. The three "galaxies" on Tammey's mammogram were cancerous tumors. Cancer is divided into stages, stage I being the least serious and stage IV the most serious. Following diagnostic tests, Tammey was diagnosed with stage IIA, which falls into the invasive cancer category. In this stage, the cancer is no larger than two centimeters in size, but it has spread to the lymph nodes under the arm; or, the cancer is between two and five centimeters in size but has not spread to the lymph nodes.

Tammey's doctor then said something Tammey had never prepared herself to hear: "You need a mastectomy."

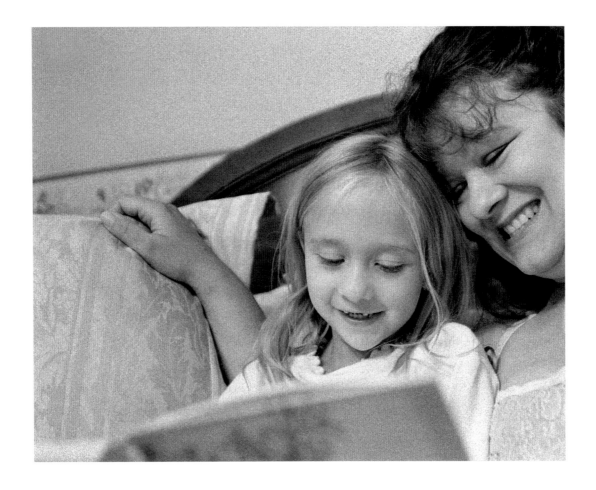

Tammey and her daughter Marie read together often. She and the children share a close bond. Throughout her illness, Tammey has been honest with her children about her cancer. "A kid's imagination is sometimes more detrimental than the truth. They make stuff up and it can be worse than what is really happening. They need to know the reality of what they are dealing with."

Tears rolled down Tammey's cheeks. She wondered if she'd heard wrong. "Why not a lumpectomy?" she asked.

The doctor told her that due to the size of the lumps and the fact there were three, a lumpectomy would deform her breast because they'd need to take out a good deal of tissue. The best route was mastectomy.

"I do not want to wake up without a breast," Tammey said. "I want the mastectomy and reconstruction done at the same time."

———

Thinking back about that day, Tammey said: "I think a woman's breasts define more than just one thing. Sexuality is one purpose, but they are also maternal. I always wanted to breast-feed my babies. I was their lifeline, their source for food. But my breasts also define me as a woman."

"I was always self-conscious. I never wore low cut stuff, but [I felt] feminine, more sexy and more sensual. My breasts not only nurture my children but also make me, as a woman, attractive to my husband because I have larger breasts."

Tammey remembered seeing a mastectomy and reconstruction operation on The Learning Channel and asked her doctor if she could have that operation. He said she could, but that operation was not done anywhere in West Virginia.

"What about the Mayo Clinic?" asked Tammey. She knew this was a top-rated clinic because her brother-in-law is a doctor there.

So the calls began, and by Monday evening, Tammey's brother-in-law scheduled her appointment for 7:30 Thursday morning.

This was what Tammey's husband Jeff called "the taking-control stage."

"The first reaction is shock," Jeff explained. "This can't happen to us. Your family is not supposed to get sick," he said, thinking back to the day of diagnosis. "I'm not one to sit around and pout. My theory is, take 15 minutes and cry and get yourself together, and then say, 'What are we going to do about it? How are we going to fix this?' We both did this. Two days later we were on a plane. All the tears were shed, and we were getting on this and fixing it."

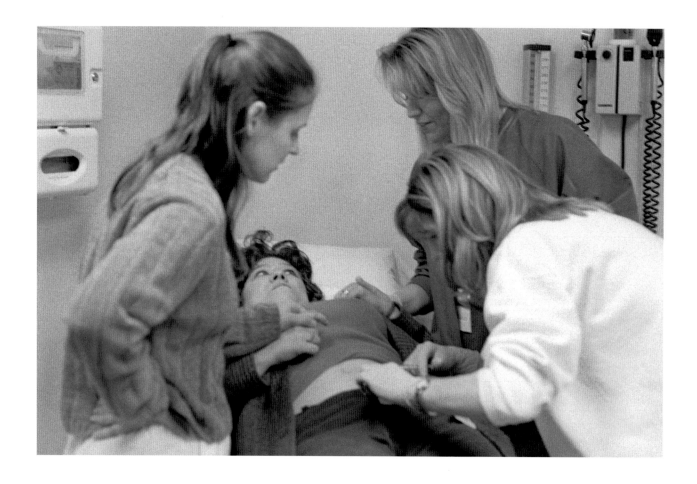

Because Tammey's cancer thrives on the estrogen her body produces, Tammey receives shots that stop the production of estrogen, sending her into menopause. Tammey was the first person to ever get this type of injection at WVU hospitals and so her treatment was a learning experience for all involved, including the Cancer Center's nurses. "Last time," Tammey says, "I started crying because the needle was so big."

The plane took them to the Mayo Clinic in Rochester, Minnesota. Tammey was listed as her brother-in-law's patient, but upon arrival was referred to one of the physicians in charge of the breast cancer center who ordered numerous tests to check for cancer outside her breast.

One by one, the tests ordered at Mayo came back normal.

"After the initial shock, the adrenaline stays there," Jeff said. "You don't feel yourself coming down. You go from test to test. How's this test result? It was good, so you go to the next. It was good. Then the surgery, it was good. You go from one success to another, and take one hill at a time."

The surgery Tammey underwent was still fairly new in 2001. The procedure was called TRAM flap, the acronym standing for "transverse rectus abdominis muscle" or, more commonly, the skin, muscle and fat from the abdomen below the navel, which is used to recreate the breast.

First, the Mayo Clinic performed a skin-saving mastectomy. Tammey's nipple and areola, the area around the nipple, were cut off and discarded. Then, all of the breast tissue was removed, leaving just the outer shell of her breast.

The plastic surgeon used a procedure similar to a "tummy tuck" to recreate her breast. All of the needed tissue, muscle, and fat from her lower stomach was cut in a football shape and stretched upward. It was tucked from underneath to fill in the shell of her breast, shaped to appear natural and then sewn into place.

Tammey's new breast appeared very natural, only missing the areola and nipple that would be reconstructed at a later time.

The procedure took close to twelve hours. Tammey's mother, father and two brothers came to Mayo for her surgery. Her sister stayed home with Tammey's children, seven-year-old Matthew and four-year-old Marie.

Resident doctors begin prepping Tammey for her nipple reconstruction. It is just after 4 p.m.

This is the second time she has come to West Virginia University Hospital for this procedure. The first time, nearly seven months earlier, Bruce Freeman, MD, chief of plastic surgery, recreated her areola using skin from her right upper thigh. He then reconstructed her nipple using half of the nipple on her left breast. This is the easiest place to use a sample from because the actual nipple is used to reconstruct the other. However, the nipple did not take hold as well as the newly reconstructed areola. This time Dr. Freeman is using the pad of Tammey's second toe to reconstruct the nipple. To make the nipple appear natural, it will need to be tattooed if the graft takes. He will also fix what Tammey calls "dog ears" on both sides of her scar from the TRAM flap operation. The "dog ears" are simply small areas of excess fat left on either side after moving the transverse rectus abdominis muscle into her breast.

The resident doctors wash her shoulders to lower stomach with warm soapy water and isolate the operation site by covering all areas they will not work on with light blue cloths. They wash her right foot where the skin graft will be removed and await Dr. Freeman's arrival.

Tammey's soft snore can be heard beneath the light blue cloth covering her face as music from the Temptations fills the room. She is still conscious and will remain so during the surgery. The anesthetic being administered is called propofol. It will keep her in a twilight state while blocking her memory throughout the surgery.

———

Tammey met with oncologist Charles Loprinzi, MD, to discuss options for chemotherapy. Although she would not remain in Minnesota for her treatments, she wanted to know what to expect. Tammey would need chemotherapy to increase her chances that cancer not recur in other parts of her body. The lymph nodes help fight infection by serving as a filter for the blood as it travels through the body and back to the heart.

According to her West Virginia University Mary Babb Randolph Cancer Center oncologist, Jame Abraham, MD, chemotherapy would increase her chance of the cancer not coming back by 80 to 90 percent.

These figures were more than enough to convince Tammey she needed chemotherapy. "If

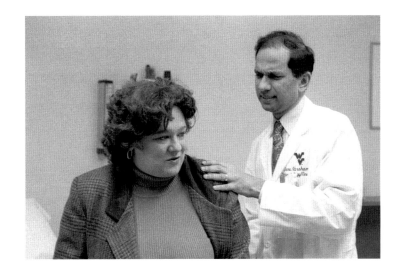

it increases my chances by that much, why wouldn't I want it?" she said. "It is my duty to do everything in my power to beat this."

She would have eight cycles of treatment, four of Adriamycin and Cytoxan, which first disrupt, then destroy cancer cells; followed by four of Taxol, which interferes with the cells during cell division. These treatments are administered intravenously though an infusaport, more commonly known as a "port," an internal central venous access device placed under the skin on her left side near her collarbone. The port can also be used to inject IV fluids and draw blood.

———

"Hey, Missy," Tammey called across her pod of cubicles in the Clarksburg office.

"What?" her sister Missy asked.

Tammey slowly ran her fingers through her highlighted, medium blonde hair, bringing out a handful of strands.

"Oh my goodness," Missy said.

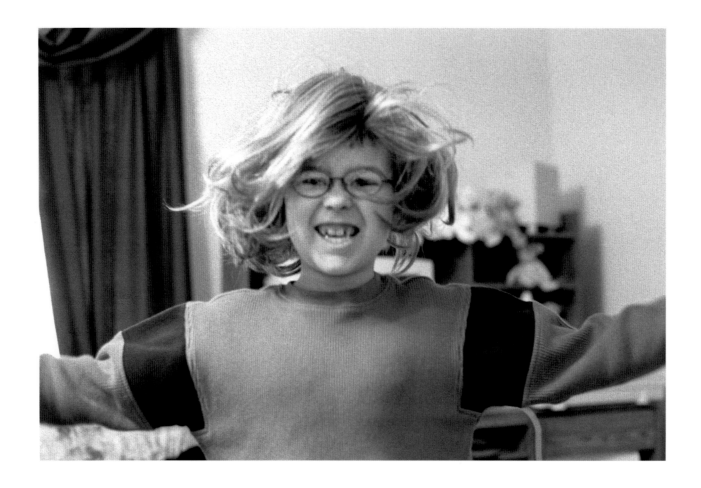

Matthew models one of the wigs his mother wore during chemotherapy treatments. According to Tammey, he is the jokester of the family. Once, despite her chronic fatigue from chemotherapy, she promised to accompany the children on a school field trip. After a particularly hectic morning rushing around to get the kids dressed, lunches made and everything packed into the family car, Tammey was unaware that she had forgotten to put on a wig for the occasion. It was Matthew who pointed out this fact. "Mom, don't you think you should wear your hair today?" he teased.

Tammey's hair was finally falling out. It horrified Missy, but Tammey joked about it because she had mentally prepared herself for this to happen.

A few weeks before beginning chemotherapy, Tammey, her mother, sister, and close friend Kelly Webster went shopping at "Chic Wigs" in Clarksburg's Meadowbrook Mall. They chose a wig by Raquel Welch. The soft blend of brown, red and blonde closely resembled her own hair color, light brown, that she had highlighted medium blonde for years. The only major difference was the length. At the time, Tammey's hair fell halfway down her back. This wig was just below chin length. Perhaps people would think she'd just gotten a haircut and added color, she told herself.

Her hair had not fallen out by the end of the first week of chemotherapy treatment. Dr. Abraham told her a small percentage of cancer patients don't lose their hair when they undergo chemotherapy.

A few days into the second week, however, Tammey's scalp began to tingle. Kelly Webster, who had battled breast cancer herself, had told her about this feeling. It was similar to what a person with long hair feels after they take a tight ponytail or barrette out of their hair. It was not a painful feeling, more of an uncomfortable one. Tammey's hair follicles were dying at the roots.

To soothe the sensation, she brushed her hair, bringing blonde strands out in clumps. Kelly had told her to use satin pillowcases when this happened because the softness of the material would help ease the sensation. She was right.

By her next chemotherapy treatment, three weeks after her first, all of her hair had fallen out. However, she began wearing a wig near the end of the second week, because her hair was thin enough to see her scalp.

When Tammey went out, she wore her wig, makeup, nice clothes and hoop earrings. She didn't want to look like a cancer patient.

"I didn't want people looking at me to know I was sick. I wanted to, I guess, masquerade my body that even though I was sick on the inside, I wouldn't look it on the outside," she said.

———

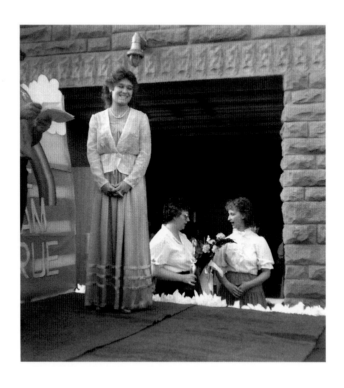

In 1981 at age 16, Tammey runs for Salem, West Virginia Volunteer Fire Department Queen. Later asked to run for Miss West Virginia Teen, she declines. "That would have required me to have a talent like singing or dancing," she muses, "but all mine were boy talents like baseball, football and sports."

On the Fourth of July, nearly four months after she had completed her treatment, she, Jeff, and the kids went to Jeff's parents' house. She went into the backyard to play baseball with Matthew and her nephew, Jimmy, who was also seven years old.

It was so hot. Sweat poured down her forehead. As she got ready to throw the ball back to Jimmy she said, "Hold on buddy," and she yanked off her wig and the nylon cap she wore underneath it.

A look of horror crossed her nephew's face. Jimmy didn't know she was sick. Jimmy didn't know she wore a wig. He thought Tammey had just gotten a hair cut and gained weight.

"You can imagine at seven years old what he thought. He thought this was his regular Aunt Tammey," said Tammey.

Throughout her battle, Tammey made sure to keep her children informed. She wanted to prevent surprises like this. She explained every step of her treatment to her children, answered every question and showed them her scars to help them understand.

"A kid's imagination is sometimes more detrimental than the truth. They make stuff up, and it can be worse than what is really happening. They need to know the reality and what they are dealing with," she said.

The Fourth was the first time she had been in public without her wig. When Tammey's hair started to grow back, she kept her wig until her hair was long enough to have somewhat of a style. When she removed her wig, dark brown, almost black, locks had replaced her light brown hair, which she had highlighted blonde for nearly 18 years. And her once-straight hair had become spiral curls.

Dr. Abraham had told her her hair would grow back another color, but he never told her about another texture. It was almost like Tammey now had completely different hair.

Texture change is the most common side effect, according to Angie Johnson, a nurse at the Cancer Center. Chemotherapy is supposed to work on cells that divide quickly, like cancer. The fastest dividing cells in the body are the cells that make up hair follicles, which is why the patient's hair falls out. But there is no exact explanation as to why cancer patients' hair grows back in differently.

Resident doctors begin numbing the areas to operate on as Dr. Freeman enters the room. The scrub nurse helps him with his gloves and ties his gown. Resident doctors stick the needle on both sides of the second toe on Tammey's right foot. She jerks her foot and gives a soft moan.

"You're going to feel a little pinch, Tammey," says one resident doctor.

"You're doing good Tammey," follows the anesthesiologist.

Dr. Freeman marks the "dog ears" with a purple marker, drawing a shape that resembles a stretched-out football with two slashes through it. He will cut along the football's outline, which is about an inch and half in length.

The resident doctors continue to numb the areas of the "dog ears" and where the nipple will be placed. Dr. Freeman draws a circle where the grafted nipple will be placed. The area is easily visible. It is light pink in color, surrounded by the tan of the grafted areola. If this graft takes hold and heals properly, both the new nipple and areola will be tattooed to match her other breast. Dr. Freeman then draws a circle on the pad of her toe to match the circle on her breast.

———

Tammey sat on the sofa in her mother's kitchen near tears. It was Christmas Day, four months into her chemotherapy and about a week into the second stage of her treatment.

"What's wrong?" her mother asked.

"I'm bald, I've gained weight, and I don't feel very attractive," Tammey answered. "I'm sick of being fat."

"Are you alive?" asked her mother.

"Yeah," Tammey answered.

"You want to be here to lose the weight don't you?" asked her mother.

"Okay, yeah, you're right," said Tammey.

"Right now you don't need to worry about that," her mother told her. "You need to get well."

Tammey understood this, but couldn't help worrying about it. She had gained between 20 and 30 pounds at this point. She couldn't fit into any of her nice clothes anymore. When she began chemo she was a size 7. At Christmas she was a 14. This was the largest Tammey had ever been.

She had worked so hard to lose weight after she gave birth to Marie four years ago and even tried to go on a diet during her treatment, but Dr. Abraham advised her it wouldn't be the best thing to do. Tammey used to think cancer patients lost weight because they were sick all the time, but she was gaining, a common side effect of chemotherapy in younger patients, according to Johnson, the oncology nurse.

———

A tourniquet is placed around her toe and held tight with an intercepts. Dr. Freeman carefully cuts along the outline of the circle and picks the graft up with tweezers. He delicately scrapes the underside of the graft to detach it from the toe. The bright yellow tissue inside the toe is exposed, and the tourniquet is removed. Blood fills the shallow hole left by the graft. Dr. Freeman blots the open toe with gauze and proceeds to sew it closed. He makes a few quick loops with the suture and ties a knot in the center of the opening. He then sews closed both sides of the opening with the same quick movements.

Freeman moves around the table to Tammey's right breast and gently scrapes the top layer of skin off the area for her nipple. Blood begins to protrude to the surface. He gently cuts along the outline of the nipple area and places the graft on, quickly sewing the left and right of the graft as blood seeps from beneath it. Freeman hopes the new nipple will attach itself to existing blood vessels and become part of the breast, which is what the first graft failed to do. He then sews the top and bottom of the graft with the same quick movements as the graft becomes outlined in blood.

———

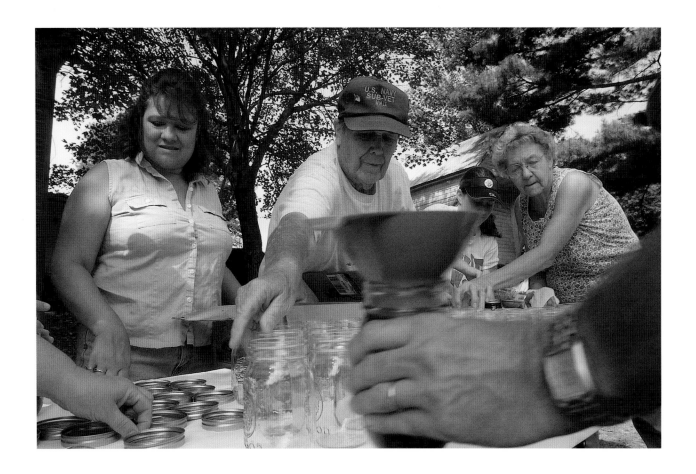

Every year at her parents' farm, Tammey makes apple butter with her "church family"—an extended group that includes close friends as well as immediate family. While she and Jeff were away for her surgery in Minnesota, the group cared for the children, sent cards and prayed for her recovery. They decorated her house with "Welcome Home" banners upon her return. "These are people you can count on," Tammey says.

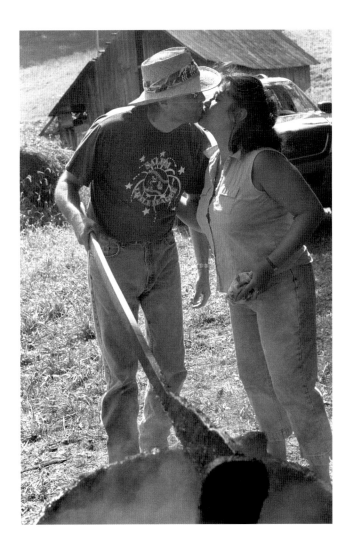

Jeff and Tammey are openly affectionate. After her surgery and chemotherapy treatments, she was hard on herself about her appearance. Tammey questioned Jeff more than once about how he could still find her attractive. "He always told me I was beautiful no matter what," she says.

"I know it's such a small part of me, but I don't feel right without it," Tammey said prior to the surgery. "I know no one knows I haven't had a nipple for the last year and half, but I know."

Tammey didn't wear her disease on her sleeve, but she knew what was going on inside her. She made the decision early in her battle not to let cancer overwhelm her life. Maintaining her appearance and piecing herself back together was one way to accomplish this, but she also needed to live her life as she had before.

———+———

Dr. Freeman begins to cut along the purple drawn lines on her side. Tammey begins to moan. The scrub nurse hands him the needle and he numbs the area again. He cuts deeper, creating an opening that spills out bright yellow tissue. Blood begins to fill the opening and is suctioned from the area. Freeman continues to cut the excess fat out. The resident doctors watch as he sews the football shaped hole back together beginning with the middle, then each side with the same quick loops as before. He returns to Tammey's right breast, places cotton over the new nipple, and ties it down with a quick knot horizontally, and then another vertically as a resident doctor finishes sewing her right side closed.

After repeating the procedure used to remove the "dog ear" on her left side, Dr. Freeman removes his gown and starts filling out a report. Resident doctors complete the sewing as Tammey gradually emerges from her twilight state.

As the anesthetics are stopped, she begins to wake up, remembering no details of the last hour and a half. The anesthesiologist asks if she has pain medicine and the nurses begin to unstrap her from the operating table. The nurses help Tammey back to the cot, and she begins to shiver as they place a white sheet on her and wheel her out of the room.

———+———

Tammey's cot is wheeled back through the thick wooden doors into a large room designated as a waiting area. There are curtains hanging from the ceiling used to designate different areas for patients, but Tammey is the only patient in the room. Nurses bring Jeff from the waiting room to see her. The last thing she remembers is leaving Jeff in the preparation area.

The sedative is quickly wearing off. As Jeff approaches she opens her tired eyes and lightly says, "Hi, Sweetie."

"I love you," he says to her.

Tammey smiles.

"I got you something from the gift shop," Jeff says as he hands her a small stuffed bear.

"Thank you, baby," she says as she looks at the bear.

One of the resident doctors who helped with her surgery approaches Tammey's cot and introduces himself before asking how she feels.

"Good," she answers.

He gives her a few general orders before she is wheeled back downstairs to the same day surgery area where she began her afternoon. She is taken into a small room with walls painted light pink on the top and darker on the bottom separated with thin trim on three sides. The entrance is divided from the main area by a glass door and a full-length window with a pastel pink and green curtain, decorated as if a painter used a thick paint brush and quick brush strokes, pulled to one side. A nurse checks her vitals and asks how she feels. Tammey has to walk with the nurse before she can leave the hospital. The nurse carries her IV bag while she accompanies her across the hallway to the bathroom. Upon their return, Tammey tells the nurse she is feeling good. The nurse checks her sides and notices they are bleeding despite being covered with tape from the surgery. She places a layer of gauze on top and uses white medical tape to secure it in place and soak up the remaining blood.

The nurse removes the IV from Tammey's port. She then sticks an L-shaped needle into the port below her collar bone and injects heparin solution to flush it. The port needs to be flushed every time it is used and about every 30 days.

After the nurse flushes her port, she leaves the room and pulls the curtain closed. Tammey changes back into her clothes and begins to put her right foot into her brown boot.

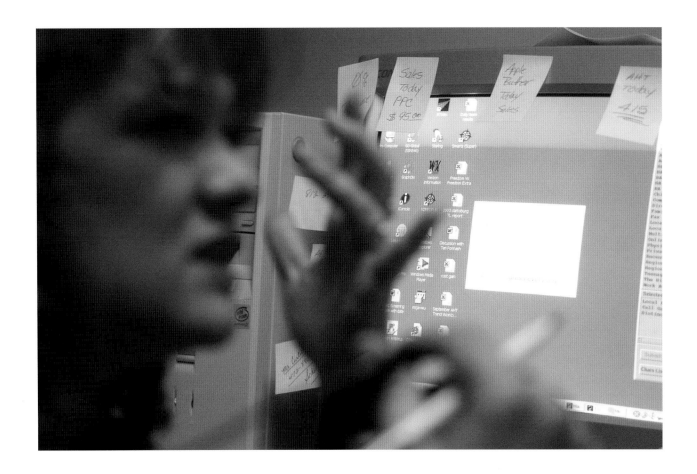

After finishing chemotherapy, Tammey noticed she couldn't remember things as well as before treatment. She started to solve the memory problem by pasting notes on her computer at work to remind her of meeting times, appointments, and important dates. "I put them everywhere," she explains. Although she still posts notes at work and home, now she carries a spiral notebook, which has become a more convenient and efficient way to keep track of her life.

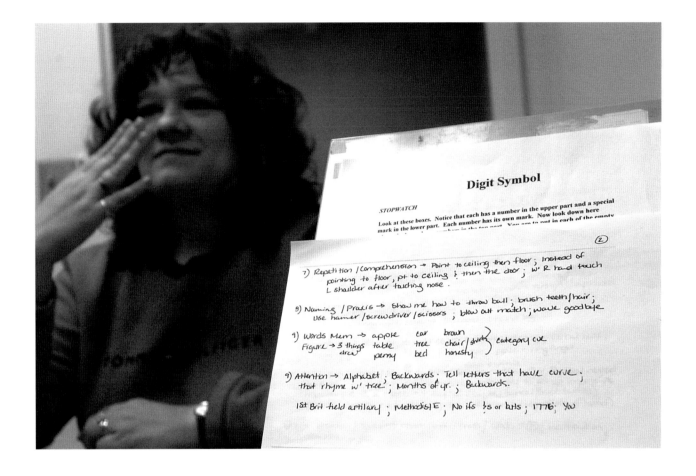

Tammey has neurological tests in Morgantown that confirm she is suffering from memory loss, for which there is no cure. The test is frustrating for Tammey, who is highly competitive and a self-proclaimed perfectionist. "I was beating myself up and found myself trying to guess the answers," she laughingly notes. "I wanted to pass that test."

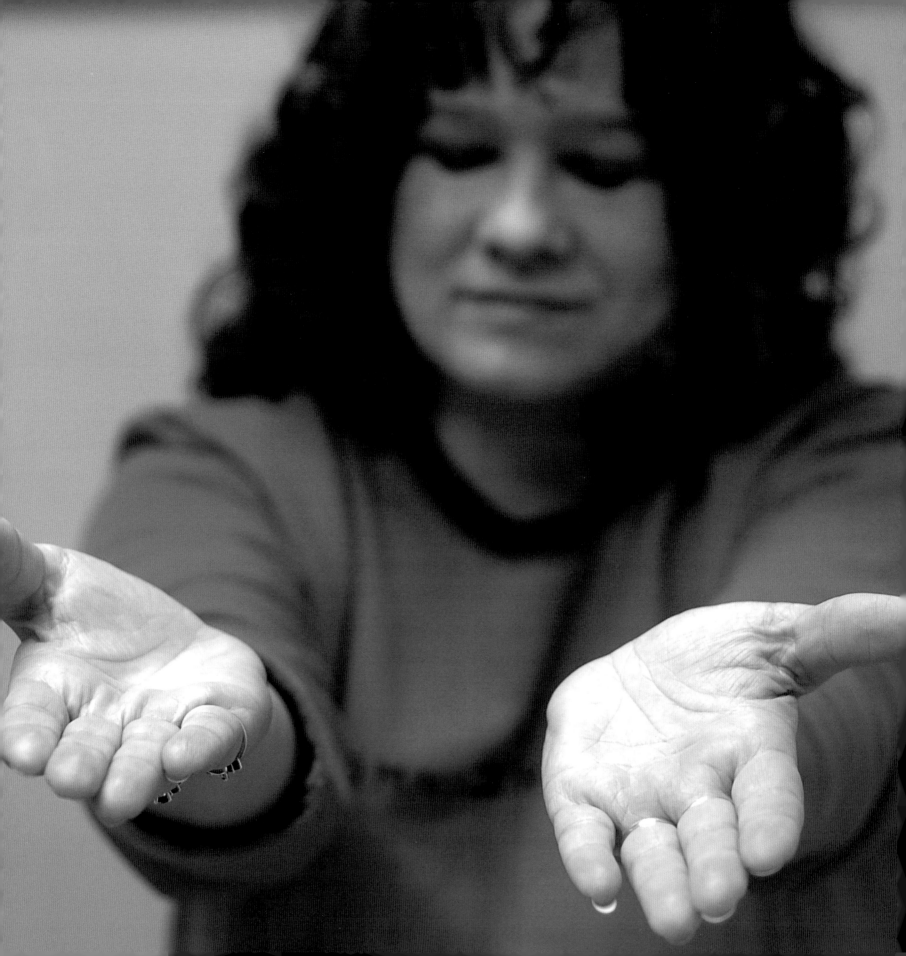

"I feel frustrated, forgetting appointments
and meetings at work. I call my kids
different names. I have forgotten my
child's football practice, and I
even forgot my own birthday party."

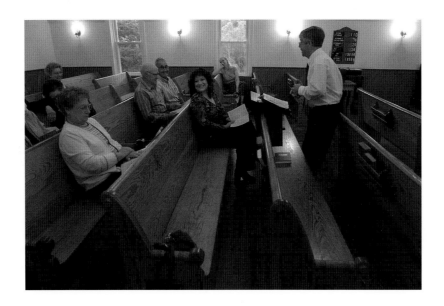

Luckily, her foot is still numb so she doesn't feel any pain when she puts weight on it. She does feel pressure, but she knows that tomorrow when she puts her shoes on it will feel much different. Jeff leaves the room to go get their dark green Explorer. After a few minutes the nurse returns with a wheelchair and wheels Tammey to the main entrance of Ruby Memorial Hospital. Jeff is waiting by the Explorer when the nurses wheel her outside, and he helps her into the front seat. After he shuts her door, Jeff walks around the back of the Explorer, climbs back into the driver's seat, and slowly pulls away from the hospital. The sun has set. It is close to seven p.m. They will reach Salem in approximately an hour and a half. In a few days, Tammey will know if the graft held. If it does, she will finally be whole again.

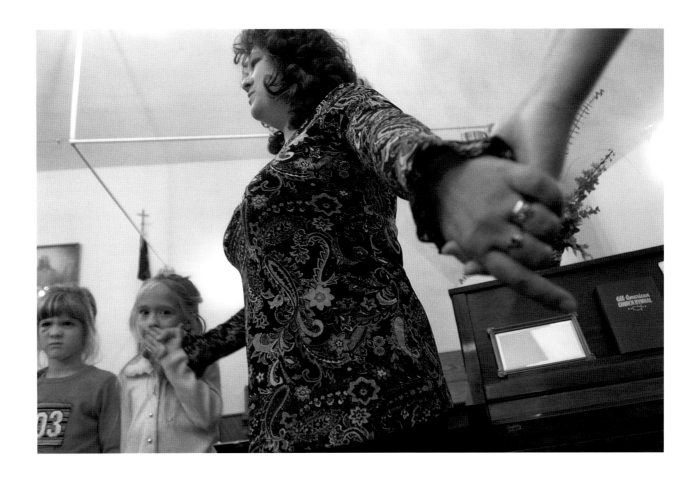

Tammey says she has become a more spiritual person since discovering that she had breast cancer. The day before she learned of her diagnosis, she had a dream that her grandmother, who died of breast cancer, sat next to Tammey along a river. "She said I would have cancer but needed to be strong for my family," Tammey says. "I just kinda put it in God's hands now."

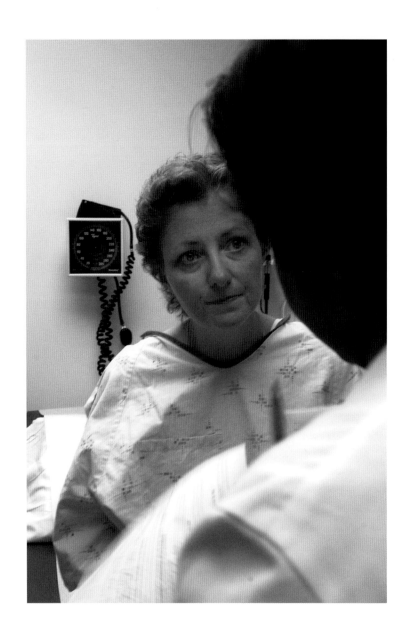

As the Legacy Descends

text by JENNIFER ROUSH

Monday

Pam Tsuhlares walks into the resort hotel—the sliding glass doors sweep out of her way—bearing a pleasant air of confidence. She hasn't looked quite as vibrant in more than a year as she does today, the day of the breast cancer event. Her blonde hair has grown back to ringlets of curls after her harshest chemotherapy treatment nine months earlier. Back then, her sister, Jody Wolfe, held a bucket for her as she vomited after each visit; now her skin glows like the juices have returned to her Irish cheeks. Tonight even her radiation doctor views her health with amazement. "Star patient" is what the doctors at the Mary Babb Randolph Cancer Center call her because she has a disease few walk away from: Stage IV inflammatory breast cancer—the most aggressive type.

Pam's oncologist, Jame Abraham, MD, had wanted to show her art ever since he heard the story behind the drawings. Human cells, bone and tissue are depicted in these pieces. Pam

---

Pam Tsuhlares listens carefully as her surgeon, Dr. Ankesh Nigam, explains the dangers and risks of the rare procedure he will perform in the hope of burning spots of cancer from her liver. Months after after undergoing a bilateral mastectomy, lymphadenectomy, chemotherapy and radiation for stage IV breast cancer, doctors have discovered the cancer has migrated to her liver.

photographs by KARINA GOMES DICK

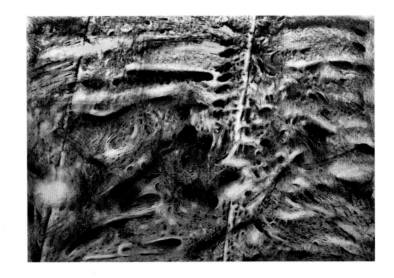

created them in the nine months before her disease was diagnosed. And she believes it's because her body knew she had cancer before she did. This event is the first time she has displayed these prophetic pieces together.

Even after enduring a bilateral mastectomy, lymphadenectomy, 12 same-day surgeries and biopsies, chemotherapy and radiation, the 44-year-old artist and mother is not yet through with her fight. She faces an approaching hurdle, a surgery on Thursday, Halloween—three days from today.

This surgery will be a laparoscopic surgery on her liver. Scorching probes will target cancer spots, which have spread to her liver. At her first consultation more than three weeks ago with her surgeon, Ankesh Nigam, MD, she signed a consent form stating that she was aware that the surgery could trigger liver failure.

"You should go home the next day," Dr. Nigam had assured Pam and Jody that day. "The reason we admit you overnight is basically for pain. Sometimes there's some pain."

"Compared to a double mastectomy and reconstruction—walk in the park," Jody had responded.

"Oh yeah, this is nothing compared to that," Pam said.

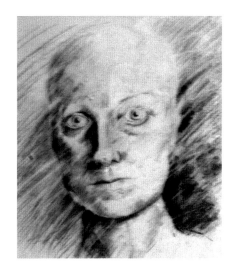

"Oh, yeah," Dr. Nigam confirmed.

Pam thought the pain couldn't be as bad as the surgery where they removed her breasts and 12 lymph nodes and reconstructed breasts out of stomach muscles they wove underneath her torso. That surgery left her looking like the "bride of Frankenstein," she'd joked, with scars crisscrossing her chest.

"I'm excited that we're able to do this," Pam had said.

"Yes, we're very glad you're going to try this with her," Jody agreed.

"I think if truly the disease is limited, and it's limited enough to be able to burn, then we have a chance of curing it," Dr. Nigam said.

The two women's faces had lit up as they heard the word "cure" used for the first time during treatment. From that day on, they expected a quick procedure and an easy recovery.

"We can do this with our eyes closed," Jody assured Pam as the nurse finished describing the pre-surgery process.

Pam was to find out that her preconceived notions about this liver surgery were wrong. Although she didn't imagine it would be as routine as when she had her ovaries removed as a precaution three months ago, she still wasn't expecting more than a few days of recovery.

However, the surgery on Halloween would turn out to be a struggle more difficult than she had ever experienced.

Pam knew cancer long before she detected a lump. The disease has shaped and reshaped her family over the generations. Her mother died of ovarian cancer more than 10 years ago. She also lost two paternal great aunts and six maternal great aunts to reproductive cancer. Pam's family history shows that her cancer is not just a scary, isolated disease. It is a worst fear come true, a deadly legacy that seems to take out every female in its genetic path. Pam's success or defeat will leave the two closest females in her life—her sister and young daughter—with hope ... or holding a ticking time bomb.

———

Jody, 49, grabs a hotel cart from the resort lobby to transport Pam's 14 pieces of art into the Cancer Center event for breast cancer survivors.

They show up on time at four p.m. But no one is there to help them, and Jody earnestly looks for someone who knows where they could set up.

"If I still had periods, I'd be having one right now," Jody says, making Pam laugh. "Well, I'm going to be proactive here." She walks up to the front-desk lady.

Jody gets things done. Her bright red hair, handful of graduate degrees and genius-level intelligence suit her do-it-yourself personality. Jody has never failed at anything, especially when it came to school. She enjoys finding patterns in data research and reading books, which line parts of her house almost everywhere you look.

"Any luck?" Pam asks as her sister comes back. They can't hang the art, but they will leave it behind the front desk.

"At least they'll be safe," Jody says.

The two make their way down the hall to a sports bar to unwind and wait for direction. Pam orders a glass of Merlot while Jody gets a bourbon and water with a twist of lemon.

"I'm about 'evented' out. This Breast Cancer Awareness Month is wearing me down," Jody says wryly, as she searches her purse for her cell phone. A nearby window shows blue skies, golf carts, and evergreens.

"In with the good air and out with the bad," Jody continues. "My problem is I've been fighting off this migraine for four days."

Today both sisters feel a bit out of sync and exhausted approaching the challenge of surgery again.

"Well, it'll be a piece of cake after this," Pam says. "You can just sit in a waiting room in the hospital. Take a good book."

"Oh yeah, nothing else to do this week except get one more surgery," Jody says sarcastically. "Although, I do a pretty good job of staying calm in the waiting room."

"You do," Pam says. "And I think actually if you look at it this way, you can't go to work. You have a good excuse for not going to work. You can't be home dealing with things. It's a time for you to have some quiet time." She laughs.

"Well this one [surgery] shouldn't be too terribly long," Jody says.

"No. I hope not," Pam trails off from the conversation to end the topic.

The sisters couldn't look or be more different. Pam is the moon, as they say, and Jody the sun.

Jody is realistic about her own chances of getting cancer. With her family history, Jody knows she most likely has the BRCA gene, a DNA mutation that inclines the possessor to ovarian and breast cancer. She never misses a mammogram or a pelvic ultrasound. In terms of prevention, Jody would prefer to have a hysterectomy but is scared of being dropped from her insurance if she tests positive for the mutated gene—a requirement to have the surgery.

Five years older than Pam, Jody has no children. But she loves animals. She has seven dogs, which make up what she calls a "fully functional dog pack." A tattoo of a wolf decorates her thigh.

Jody spins off witty quips, while Pam is a thoughtful storyteller. Pam has always been the artistic one with spiritual insights. She keeps journals and enjoys exploring different realms of thought in her artwork. One of Pam's favorite places is sitting on her porch with a cup of tea as a beam of sun cuts through the tree in her front yard, hitting her face as the wind rustles through her wind chimes.

Pam and Jody both studied at West Liberty State College in Wheeling, West Virginia, and

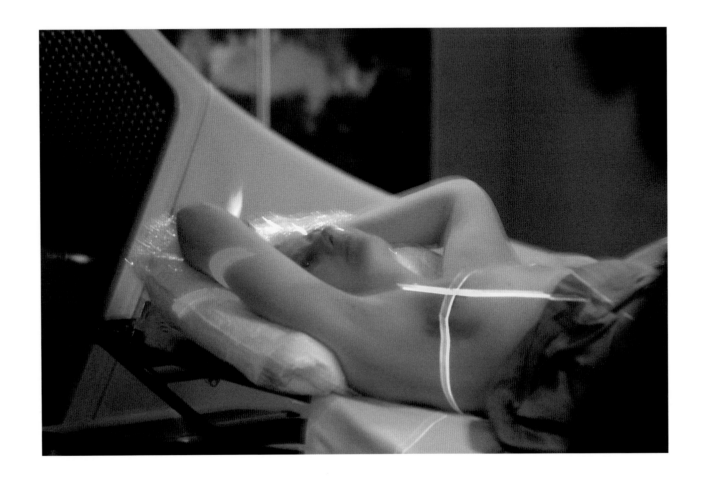

Pam undergoes radiation therapy at Ruby Memorial Hospital, West Virginia University. Photos by Jason DeProspero

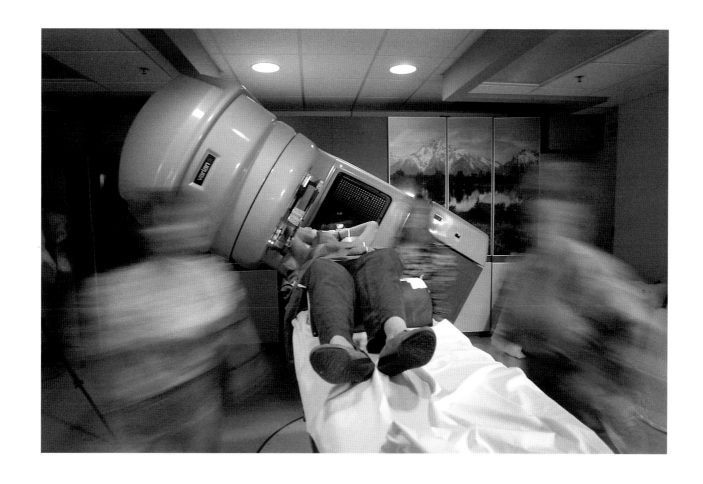

remained close throughout their lives. Pam enjoys books too, but instead of data research, she channels her energy into finding a peace that will help her get in touch with the spiritual realm and God. Her beliefs are rooted in Christianity. But now, being out of the church, she feels art is a way God can work through her.

This evening Pam is wearing loose artist's clothes that are good for working with paint but also a bit earthy in color and style. Jody wears black attire with pearl earrings and a matching necklace she bought in Las Vegas.

Soon, Pam's art stands on tables inside the large ballroom. The lighting is dim, and a single candle flickers on each table. Doctors, donors and survivors can hear a harp in the background. The atmosphere at the benefit is strangely reminiscent of the radiation room, with its soft music and low lighting. Last summer, Pam had daily dates with the radiation machine, which hovered around her exposed chest, as her arms were positioned above her head on a solid Styrofoam pillow.

Now, people lean over the pink, cloth-draped tables to get a closer look at Pam's charcoal drawings. Most stares become blank expressions—with conversations limited to whispers—as they browse the corner display.

"They speak for themselves," Pam tells Jody.

The first drawing is Pam's self-portrait when she was bald from chemo. She originally thought it would be funny to call herself "egghead." However, after the sunken eyes and empty gaze emerged, Pam chose to call it "Self-portrait as the Legacy Descends." A figure drawing of a young girl follows and then her "egg drawings" and her "spirit drawings." The egg drawings depict an egg placed next to a wall, and as they progress it seems as if a spirit pierces through it. The spirit drawings arose from the evolution of the eggs, where Pam drew what appeared to be faces in a spiritual essence.

Another dramatically different series of pictures Pam calls the "bone drawings." The largest piece in this series stands in a hollowed-out section of the wall with a lone light shining upon it, like a frightening apparition waiting to jump out of the darkness. The black-and-white drawing seems to be a microscopic view of cells, bone marrow and tissue impaled on a spinal cord. Jody still can't stand to look at this drawing. However, Pam is no longer afraid of it—this first picture that started it all—the one that foreshadowed her deadly disease.

Two years ago, long before she was diagnosed with cancer, Pam lived as an artist and piano teacher in a little blue house in Wheeling, where she still lives today. Her husband Lambros, a tall Greek-American man, had worked at a pottery studio a few miles away. Three children scrambled in and out of the house, carrying book-bags and baby dolls. Ana, Lambros' daughter from a previous marriage, stayed with them throughout the year and lived with her mother in the summer. John, Pam's son from a previous marriage, stayed with his father on and off but lived with Pam. Lambros and Pam's daughter, Joey, was only two at the time, and Pam had little time for her artistic work, and most of that time came at night.

Breast-feeding and tending to a baby for two years, Pam rarely felt the urge to draw. So when a concept emerged from a drawing in her sketchbook, she would pursue it.

In the kitchen, with jelly still stuck to the countertop and the smell of the evening's dinner lingering in the air, Pam found a place to get away—her own personal artistic retreat. She had to find a time to be alone where children weren't asking her for a glass of orange juice or to look for a missing sock.

One night, insomnia caused Pam to toss and turn in bed with her mind racing. Her head was filled with images she could not escape. Being a mother with a young demanding toddler was draining. But the images were persistent, and finally she shook off the reality that she needed rest to get her kids ready for school the next morning and decided to draw. She gently pulled the covers away so as not to wake up her sleeping husband. And with a creak and a pause, her feet hit the cold floor. She sneaked down the stairs, trying not to wake the kids.

Pam picked up a broken piece of charcoal and listened to her instincts. She believed her insights came from a higher power—God would guide her.

In the dark of night, with charcoal smudges on the side of her right hand, she pulled back her waist-length blond hair and drew, not knowing what the black markings on white paper represented.

She was frightened of her creation. "What is this?" she asked herself.

Before, she drew eggs and human portraits, but this was flesh, human cells, and bones. The picture appeared on the paper before her section-by-section, like it had already been there, and she was just pulling it out.

Drawing two pictures simultaneously to get out all of her pent-up creativity, Pam sighed and looked around. She often drew this way, sometimes calling it "sounding," a term used for whales when they dive deep into the ocean. She dove deep into herself. She knew instinctively this experience had been different from the way she normally developed an idea. This was something that was truly emerging from her very bones.

She raised her head and felt dread. What if this image were trying to tell her something?

———

Over the next few weeks, her inspiration continued. Pam continued to develop the two drawings, and she felt satisfied with her creations. Pam let her friend, Cece, look at the main drawing as it developed.

"I hope this isn't something growing inside of me," Pam joked, choking back a deep fear.

She even had a physician—the father of one of her piano students—give his professional opinion.

"Rex, look at this," she said. "What does this look like?"

"Well," the doctor said, "it seems close up like it's some kind of soft tissue or bone marrow."

Nine months later, she found her worst fears confirmed when she felt a lump during a self-exam—a tumor.

———

In the weeks before the breast cancer event, the sisters' routine had been interrupted. Before, when Pam had an appointment, she traveled an hour and a half to Morgantown and usually stayed overnight at Jody's home a few miles from the Cancer Center. That was becoming their weekly routine, and Pam's daughter Joey was a part of it. But Pam had recently begun taking a chemo pill that was her ticket to a normal life again, giving her the freedom to stay at home. Now the sisters had hope that they were approaching a miraculous surgery, a miracle because there weren't many more options to stop Pam's disease. The hope continued to be that they would come to the end of this cancer. And that end would begin with the surgery on Halloween.

During their time apart, Pam fully returned to the mom role, and Jody caught up on work at *Woofs*, her dog supply and grooming shop.

Pam's healthy appearance was deceiving, especially with demanding children aged 4, 11 and 12. Pam was stronger than she had been since she was diagnosed, and the blood test for her tumor marker was down, so the chemo was working. The world was making sense again.

"It's not usually done, but there have been people who have done it for breast cancer. I don't know of the results," Dr. Nigam told Pam and Jody at her appointment three weeks ago. "We're not exactly sure what we're going to find. There's a small possibility it's not a tumor—that would be the best thing. And then, if that's not true, we'll at least biopsy it and prove that it is. And if there's limited disease, then we can try to burn it."

But now they are back, back in Morgantown and at an event, which brings them back to reality: Pam is sick and still a cancer patient. And these next three days will bring challenges. Although they are both thankful for the surgery, it is still a risky and rare procedure.

———

Her mind elsewhere, Pam claps softly as a cancer survivor steps down from the podium inside the resort. The cheery, pink environment and uplifting testimonies of the women didn't change the looks on Pam and Jody's faces. They are sympathetic, but their focus is somewhere else. The team is mentally preparing for the next round.

They wait until the crowd clears out before they take down the drawings and load them back into Jody's RAV4.

"That was pretty painless," Pam says as she finishes packing her art.

They have a long three days ahead of them. For her surgery the doctors will try a procedure the hospital has performed only a couple times. But this may be the only hope.

They have been through harder times and worse surgeries, the sisters convince themselves. They are cancer treatment veterans.

Six months earlier during a chemo treatment, Pam and Jody thought they had been through

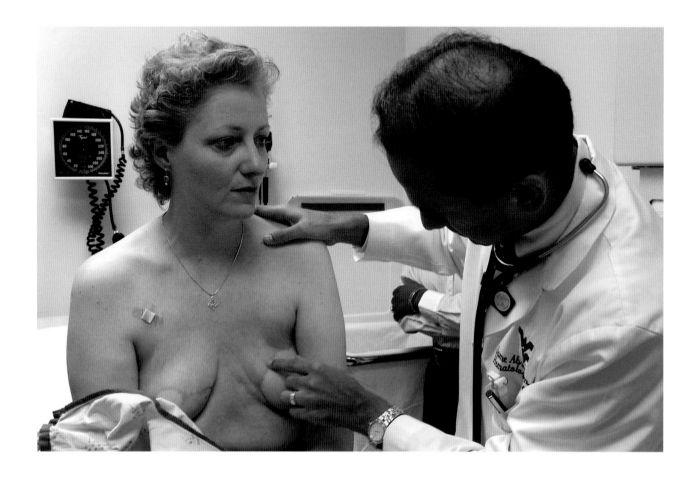

During a routine checkup months after surgery, her oncologist, Dr. Jame Abraham, examines Pam's breasts while they talk about how she has been feeling. It was during one such regular appointment that he found a red spot on her chest, an indication that Pam's breast cancer had reccurred, spreading to the lymphatics of her skin.

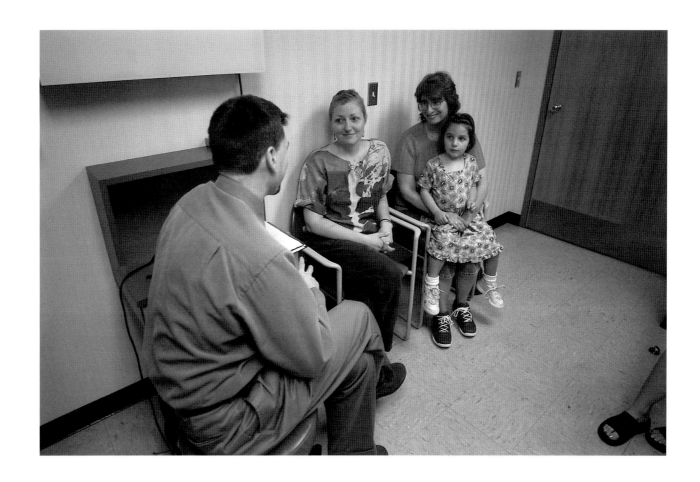

A radiation oncologist updates Pam, sister Jody and daughter Joey on her treatments. Because the tumor was close to her heart, doctors had to proceed with caution. For each appointment, Jody is there with love and support.

Photo by Jason DeProspero

the hardest part of cancer. The cancer in Pam's breasts and lymph nodes was removed, and doctors had reconstructed her breasts. If all went well, they would add an implant to make the left breast look more even and then surgically tattoo on nipples.

But then, during a regular appointment with Dr. Abraham, he informed them that a red spot on Pam's chest was a reccurrence of her cancer. Pam's breast cancer had spread to the lymphatics of her skin, which caused the spot, a blemish on the "clean slate" that Dr. Abraham had given her after surgery.

Her chemotherapy cycle was halted, and she was scheduled for radiation oncology where they would target the spot and the most vulnerable places on her chest.

After the doctor left the patient room that day, the sisters had looked at each other.

"Well, that's it," Jody had assured Pam. "We just need to nip it in the bud right now."

"Yeah. Yeah," Pam said. "Well, that's what I was afraid of."

The sisters sat, Pam in a green gown that was becoming far too familiar, and Jody in the seat designated for a loved one. They looked at each other and moved past the shock straight to a solution.

"We can do this," Jody said.

"We can do this," Pam confirmed.

"This can't be as bad as chemo," Pam said.

"Oh, don't say that. Shut your mouth," Jody joked.

TUESDAY

The day after the breast cancer event, Pam wakes up at Jody's house. It's her home away from home in Morgantown, which houses the top cancer treatment center in the state. The window in front of her room in the cabin-like house forecasts the day for her—wet, gray and windy.

It isn't beautiful like the view she came home to after she was released from the hospital following the surgery that transformed her breasts. But almost nothing would be.

Back in January, she had returned from losing her breasts to a winter scene of snow-dusted trees out the window, a warm cup of tea and a sublime sense of accomplishment.

Today, in the same room, Pam doesn't see the same perfect day out the window. It's a bit dismal to take Joey and her two-year-old friend Brenlynn to have professional pictures taken. However, the rainy weather outside is not enough to dampen her daughter's thrill at being made up like a doll.

Making up Joey for the pictures takes no coercing. The young Greek-Irish girl looks in the bathroom mirror without a passing glance at the world around her. Her Aunt Jody and her mom wrap her long brown hair around a curling iron to form ringlets, which tumble down her black and red-plaid dress.

Holding her daughter's hair in her hands, Pam remembers and wants to believe Joey's words from a couple months ago: "When your hair grows back, you don't have to go to the doctor anymore," she said to her mom after Pam finally had enough hair to fix again.

"Look at that hair," Pam says, releasing a curl that falls next to Joey's face. "It's beautiful."

"So, how should we do this? What should we do first?" Pam asks Joey.

"The back," Joey responds.

"Or the front? Maybe some curls down the side?" Pam asks. "Because she's got these short pieces from when we C-U-T H-A-I-R."

Pam picks up a short curl of her hair and sighs, remembering how that happened. It started with Pam losing her hair.

———

PAM'S JOURNAL MARCH 12, 2002:
One should be able to feel like a woman, and I feel all that has (at least temporarily) been stolen.

A year and a half earlier, a continuous flow of water sprayed Pam's back in her small upstairs shower. She put shampoo in her hand and lathered it to clean her long, blond mane. The beauty of her hair flowing over her small frame is what caught the eye of her husband Lambros

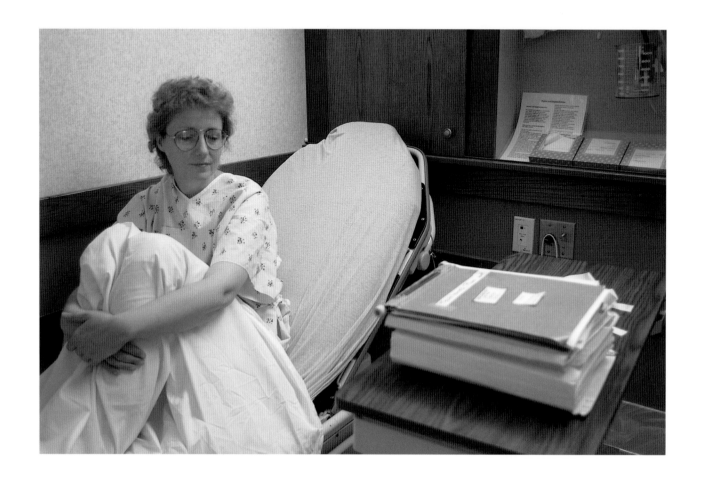

Pam's file grows bigger as she prepares for another surgery. Pam has undergone 12 same-day surgeries, chemotherapy and radiation treatments—in addition to the surgery that removed her breasts and lymph nodes. This time, Dr. Nigam will try a laparoscopic surgical technique using new laser technology in an attempt to remove cancer spots from her liver.

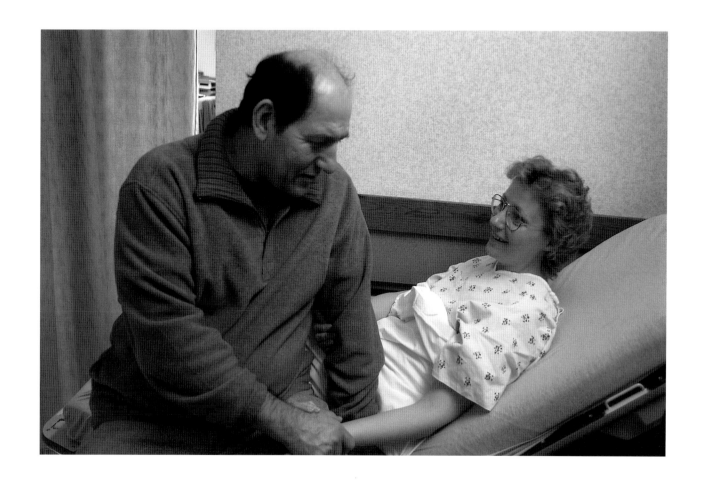

Moments before going into surgery, Pam and her husband Lambros share a close moment. As much as she looks relaxed, they're both acutely aware that the procedure is a delicate and risky attempt at eradicating the cancer.

in the art class where they met. Pam never intended to cut her hair short. But here in the shower it was falling out in clumps in her hand. The shower of water became a shower of hair, covering her pale skin. She realized she had to stop living in denial. Her hair had to come off.

The next morning Pam walked into her bedroom with a devastated look on her face, and she couldn't hide being upset from her husband.

"Let's just do it. Let's just get it over with," Lambros said while comforting her.

Pam agreed it was time.

"Leave us alone for a while," they told Ana, John, and Joey before they locked themselves inside the bathroom.

Pam stared at her head, already showing patches of her scalp. Lambros took the razor, and they couldn't help but laugh through it.

As the last lock of hair fell, the couple looked at each other in the mirror. The person looking back at Lambros was his new wife—his new wife who visibly had cancer.

Pam walked out of the bathroom and said, "Hey kids, come here, look at this."

She wanted to be honest with the kids and let them know this is just something that happens—anything to keep them from being afraid of her baldness. She thought if she was normal about it, then they would be too.

The kids laughed and touched her bare scalp.

Joey soon found an opportunity to sneak off with a pair of scissors. She decided she wanted to cut her hair off too. She grabbed a large chunk of waist-length brown hair from the top of her head and snipped it off. Pam found her in her room just in time; she had cut only the top.

———

In Jody's bathroom mirror, Pam stares back at her little girl as she curls her hair, laughing to herself about that time when her daughter said she wanted to be like her.

Joey stands perfectly still letting her mom fix her hair. Jody helps apply hairspray and looks for the perfect clips to put final touches on her hair. With two heart-shaped rhinestone clips snapped, she's ready to have her picture taken.

The last surviving women in Pam's family, except for one great aunt, stand together in the bathroom. The legacy of cancer haunts every female in their family bloodline—including Jody and Joey. They will both have to live with it in the back of their minds—"Is it going to happen to me?"

The frightened eyes in Pam's self-portrait show her inner fear. She looks unsure about why this had to happen to her and when it is going to stop.

Pam won't even fully articulate her fear for Joey. She hopes scientists find a cure by then. That thought simmers in her subconscious as she continues to hope for a better life for her daughter.

WEDNESDAY

The day before surgery, Joey sits on her makeshift bed, which is actually a big chair at Jody's house. She jumps up and grabs on to her mom's single bed to climb up. She likes to be right by her mom, so she can whisper secrets to her or give her spontaneous kisses and hugs. Joey has darker skin like her dad and a mature face with prominent features. She's tall for a girl her age, and smart.

"Joey says that Grandma speaks to her heart," Pam says.

Pam picks up a picture of her mother as a young girl, and the image is almost identical to Joey. Pam looks at the picture and is taken back to more than ten years ago, when her mother was diagnosed with ovarian cancer, and when she got the news that her mother was going to die.

When the doctor called Pam, she and her mother were sitting across from each other at a round table in her old house in Wheeling. Her mother was on the phone extension and looked at her daughter through large plastic-framed glasses with stark, thinning black hair as they both received the news of the sonogram. The doctor didn't know her mother was on the line.

"It's terminal. It's invaded the entire abdominal cavity. There are spots on the liver, and we think it's in the lungs. There's a mess here. There's nothing we can do," the doctor said. "Do you want me to tell your mother or do you want to do it?"

Many such scenes live in Pam's subconscious from those last three months as she watched her mother deteriorate. Back then, Pam did for her mother what Jody is now doing for her. She sat next to her when she was sickest. Pam laughed and talked to her mom, a lot like she and Jody do. Her mom taught her how to sustain grace during tough situations. Pam knew she was the one who'd be with her as she chose how to die. She had to get a grip on the situation and not lose control.

The day her mother died, Pam sat on her mother's bed and took her hand. Her mother's long, bony fingers wrapped around Pam's, and they intertwined their fingers over and over. They kept holding hands, not wanting to let go.

Pam's visual memory and total recall were going to be a curse to her, she thought as she sat there a few hours before her mother died, because she was going to remember what it all looked like—her face, her fingers and her illness.

Pam has clear, vivid pictures of the horror of the disease and the dying. She doesn't want to remember that as clearly as she does.

Joey had never met her Grandma, who died before she was born. Pam's family lineage stares at both of them as they rest on Pam's guest bed—grandparents, great grandparents, and many others, occupy frames captured in black and white images.

Pam looks at her little girl beside her on the bed and asks her about the times she said she hears from her grandparents.

"When does Grandma talk to you?" Pam asks.

"When I'm asleep," Joey says staring down at the toy in her hands. "She says, 'Keep doing it.' Grandpa says, 'Keep playing.'"

"That sounds like something my mother would have said," Pam says.

———

Joey has gone through phases with her mom's illness. She'd been with her mom through most of her treatment.

When Pam lost her hair, out of the three kids, her mom's bald head continually fascinated only Joey, and she was two. She grabbed at Pam's scarves and wanted to feel her head.

That was until Joey started to figure it out. Her mom being bald meant that she was sick. She had to see doctors and go away to hospitals.

Her understanding of the cancer emerged at the most shocking times.

Several months earlier, in the same bathroom where Pam curled Joey's hair, Joey revealed to her aunt Jody for the first time that she understood the severity of her mom's disease. Jody was bathing Joey in her large, round jet bathtub. Pam was sick and recovering from a surgery in her bedroom at Jody's house. Joey, three at the time, scooted a bath toy in the bubble-filled tub and looked up to Jody with her large blue eyes. "You know my grandma died," she said.

"Yes, Joey, I know that," Jody said.

"Is my mama going to die?" Joey asked.

"We certainly hope not," Jody responded

"But she's sick, and when my grandma got sick, she died," Joey said.

"Yes, your mommy's sick, but sometimes when you're sick you get well and we're working on trying to get your mommy well again," Jody said. "Usually what happens is that people live a very, very long time, and they get to be very old, and then they get sick and die."

Joey sat in the bath, thinking about that idea. That answer made sense to her for the time being. She nodded "OK," and continued playing in the suds.

"And if anything happens you'll always have your daddy, you'll always have me, and you'll always have Uncle Ray [Jody's husband]," Jody said. "We'll always be right here with you."

———

For Halloween this year, Joey is going to be a princess-witch.

While Pam is at her pre-surgery appointment the day before the surgery, Joey gets to hang out at Woof's and help Megan, the groomer, wash and brush the dogs.

"Hi, Joey," the shop owners say to the smiley girl as she whispers a reply. Even though she acts shy sometimes, she loves the camera, dressing up and being in pictures. She has her own fantasy world with horses, dragons, and fairy tales.

Joey stands on a stool and watches Megan put the shampoo on a big pug dog named Lucy.

Sometimes she'll help brush after they are dry, but she mostly watches. After she finishes with Lucy, Joey runs into the store and finds a place to sit.

When someone calls her a big girl, Joey says, "I don't want to grow up."

Joey says this often, sometimes revealing the reason: when you grow up, you die. In her own world, she can avoid the big problems. She can find a game in anything. Sitting on the floor, she takes a little bag of Halloween Sweet-Tarts and plays with them. She's quiet and introverted, but in her eyes you can see she knows a lot.

However, Joey thinks the hospital is a good place for her mom to be. She knows that's where she gets better.

Later in the evening, Joey gets into her Halloween role in Jody's living room, which has a cathedral ceiling. Joey has the princess role down—she dresses in princess gowns even when it's not a holiday.

Her mom needs to make alterations to the costume. It is purple, Joey's favorite color, with sheer layers of purple and pink as the skirt, and purple sequins on top. Pam puts the dress on Joey with a white turtleneck underneath, so she is warm. *Free Willy* plays in the background. Pam sees the dress is too long. She takes a pair of scissors and cuts it jagged to make the dress more "witchy" for her princess-witch ensemble.

Joey takes the pieces Pam cuts off and gently places them on Pam's head as she finishes cutting.

"It makes you look pretty," Joey says. Pam smiles and takes the pieces, braids them and puts them around Joey's pointy witch hat.

"You are going to be the most beautiful princess-witch," Pam says.

Joey dances in her costume and says she wants to wear it all day. Pam talks to her about the surgery tomorrow, as she always does, to prepare Joey for her being sick and to assure her that the surgery will help her.

"I'm going to have booboos," Pam says to Joey.

"Why?" Joey says in her not-accepting-a-serious-talk tone. She continues to dance as the light jumps through the glass doors to the back porch. Pam sighs and continues putting the pieces away.

The two have become inseparable. Joey is attached to Pam's hip; however, the two depend on each other equally.

"Joey, you going to save me treats tomorrow?" Pam asks.

"Yep," Joey answers.

"Chocolate," Pam specifies.

The dogs erupt in ear-splitting cacophony. Jody is home with bags of groceries in her arms. Joey perks up at the prospect of a new person.

"Oh, it's just Jody," she says.

"I've loaded up on man-friendly food," Jody says. The two women will be at the hospital, leaving Ray and Lambros with Joey. Jody also picked up a Dracula costume for whichever of the two men will take Joey trick-or-treating.

"Oh, you got Pringles. I can't eat. I can't eat." Pam reminds herself as she throws her arms up and shakes her head.

"Oh, I'll get you whatever you want tomorrow night," Jody replies sympathetically.

It's time now for Pam to take her pre-surgery medication, which is a powerful laxative so she won't have anything in her bowels during her surgery. Pam accepts that she will be in the bathroom for an hour and heads upstairs with a bottle of water, a Sprite and a cup.

Joey plays with blocks as her Aunt Jody balances her checkbook. Tonight Joey is on a make-believe farm. Wearing her fairy-princess dress, she fits blocks together. She has a distant look in her eyes, like she's trying not to think. Like she's just trying to create another world on the ottoman with her blocks that she says are baby sheep and mama cows.

THURSDAY: SURGERY DAY

The next day, at 5:35 a.m., gravel crumbles as Lambros turns his old white covered-bed truck into Nettie's driveway. Nettie watches Joey for Pam when she goes to Morgantown for her treatments. Joey calls her "Grandma Nettie."

Lambros walks around to the passenger side and picks up his sleeping daughter. She partially opens her eyes as he cradles her, blanket and all. He makes sure she's covered by the pink, patched blanket and walks up the stairs in the morning's silence and darkness.

Pam follows them. She is weak from only eating a couple pieces of deli-sliced turkey the evening before and then being up most of the night from the laxative.

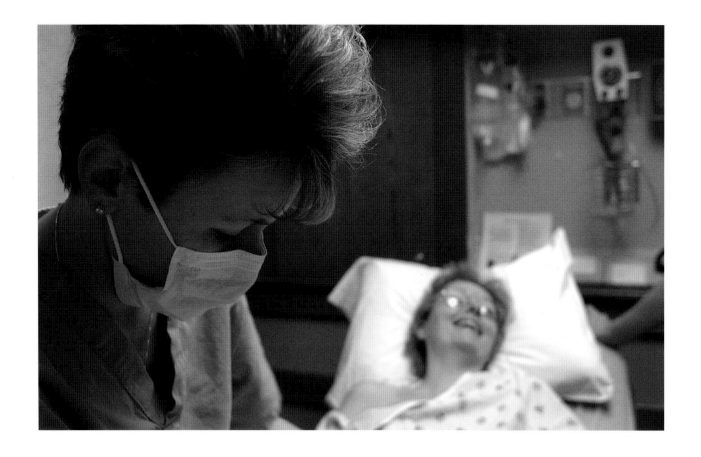

Prepping for surgery, Pam tries to maintain a good sense of humor as Jody tells her a joke. But minutes later, she will be in pain again as the nurse has a difficult time finding Pam's port. In the end, another nurse comes to her assistance.

Nettie opens the screen door, which whines every inch of the way until the trio makes its way through the door, and then she closes the door with them as they walk in, like tucking them into bed.

They greet each other softly as Lambros places Joey on the couch where she will sleep the rest of the morning. Even though they whisper, Joey wakes.

"Can you give your mom a big hug and kiss?" Pam asks, and then she squeezes her. "I love you."

Pam holds onto her daughter a little longer than normal, catching the scent of her hair as her head rests on her shoulder in the embrace.

"I want to kiss you," Joey says to Pam.

"Okay," Pam says as Joey wraps little arms around her mother's neck and kisses her.

"You go back to bed and have one of those nice dreams with the sparkles in it," Pam says.

"I want to talk to daddy," Joey says, and then she whispers in her dad's ear.

Pam explains to Nettie that Joey hasn't seen Lambros in a few days. They chat while father and daughter have a secret conversation.

"Good-bye. I love you," Pam repeats until she is sure Joey believes it and remembers it.

"I love you," Pam says.

Lambros kisses Joey on the head, and he and Pam walk away, breaking the silence with each step in that quiet, dark autumn morning.

The desk calls for "Tsuhlares," and Lambros and Jody rise out of their waiting room seats in Ruby Memorial Hospital without a word. They have been waiting several hours. Now it is just a walk to the back, to the intensive care unit (ICU) to see Pam. They already know Pam is OK.

The surgery was a success. Dr. Nigam came out earlier and drew a diagram showing them how they burned a large part of Pam's liver—more places than they knew she had. Dr. Nigam burned all the cancerous spots on her liver.

Jody is in dedicated, proactive-sister mode. She remains cautiously optimistic, as her facial expression remains locked on concern.

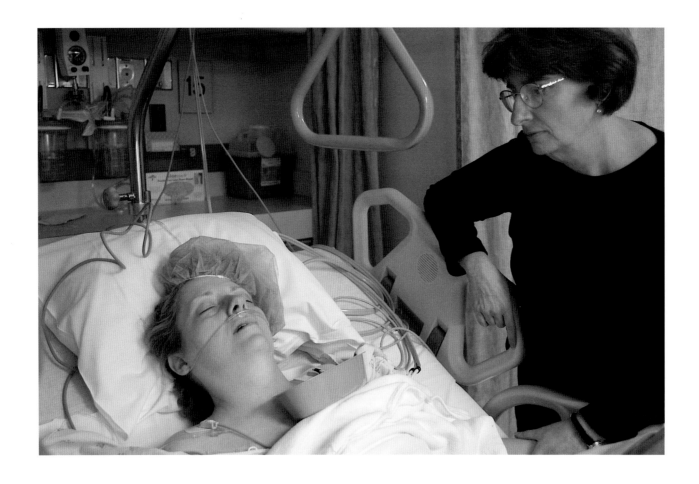

In the ICU minutes after liver surgery, Pam squeezes Jody's hand, acknowledging her presence. After all the surgeries and many hospitalizations, the sisters have come to understand the gesture as meaning "it's over, and I am OK."

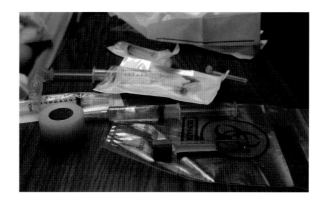

They wheel Pam on a bed into the ICU as doctors attempt to speak to her. Barely conscious, she manages to ask for her sister. Pam can't do anything about the fiery pain in her stomach as the anesthesia wears off, except to hope that relief arrives soon. She lies stiff and motionless because moving makes the pain even more intense. Surrounded by green curtains, she waits for her family.

Walking back through ICU is brisk. There is no lagging. Halloween pumpkin and ghost pictures decorate a desk near the flapping double doors. Nurses' eyes follow the two as they enter the place where patients recover from going under the knife.

In the ICU, green-scrubbed surgeons, nurses, and anesthesiologists bustle around an island of data and statistics that only the professionals understand. The nurse pulls back the sheet-like curtain unveiling Pam, barely conscious and not yet stable.

Her face can't even grimace in pain yet; it hurts her too much to move. The doctors said it'd be painful; they burned a large part of her liver. But not much can prepare a husband and sister to see their beloved in this state. Just eight hours ago she was well and cracking jokes. Now she can barely croak, "It hurts," as doctors scramble for pain medication.

Pam is moving. She holds on to Lambros' arm and Jody takes the other hand. Pam's lips are laced with black, dried blood from when the oxygen tube was pulled from her throat. She is more pale than usual, and she can't open her eyes except for an occasional squint, which takes all of her strength. A drool cup is placed under her chin, as Lambros stands to the right and Jody to the left of Pam.

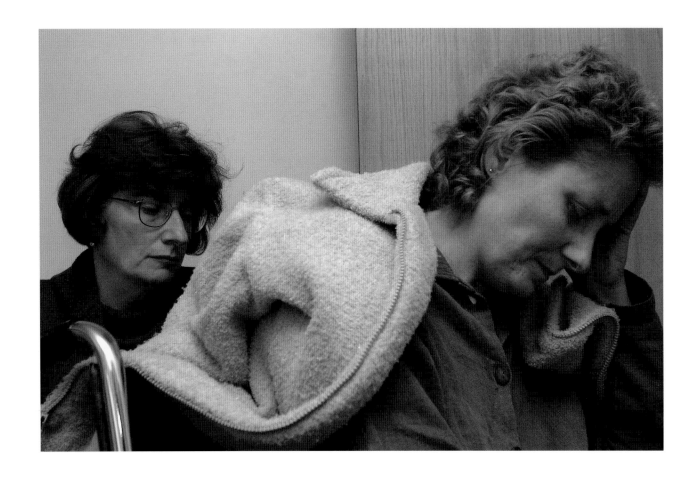

Just a few days after her liver surgery, Pam and Jody are back in the hospital. Pam complains about severe pain and asks to be readmitted. The surgery is causing side effects, and doctors want to keep her under observation.

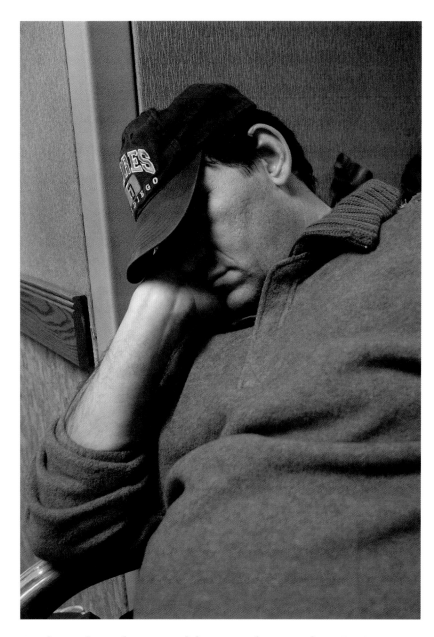

Lambros takes a short nap while waiting for news about Pam's surgery. The tension is so great that he wakes with a start every half hour. Waiting is an all-too-familiar reality for everyone involved.

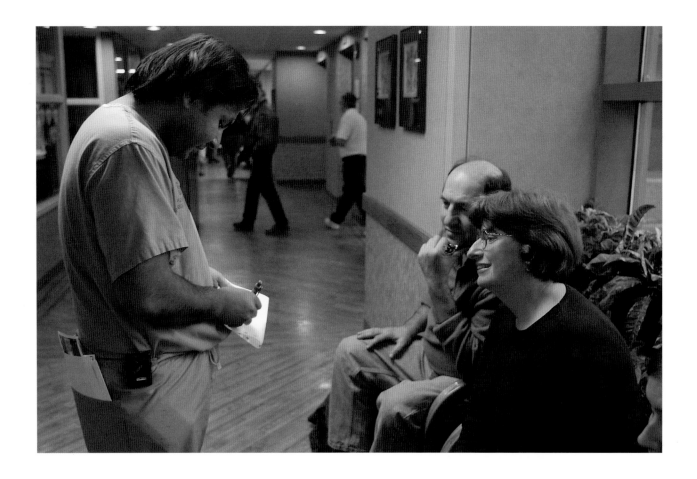

After waiting for more than five hours, Jody and Lambros listen to Dr. Nigam as he draws a diagram showing them how doctors burned a large part of Pam's liver—there were more spots than the doctors anticipated. In addition to scorching all the cancerous spots on her liver, he removed her gallbladder because it had been burned. After a few nervous moments, they smile in relief as he reassures them that the surgery went as well as expected.

Jody is calm as she holds tightly to her sister's clammy hand. It looks as though Pam has lost ten pounds, with her darkened eyes and weak movements. Jody remains strong, like she is trying to do it for the both of them. She gazes at her sister from behind her glasses without a change in expression and pets Pam's hand, barely raised above the bed.

And there is silence, no soothing words and no humor, just silence. Pam can't even intertwine fingers with Jody—they just hold on.

The doctors gave her morphine, a drug that makes Pam nauseated and ill. Jody forgot to tell them about her reactions to pain meds. The morphine makes her condition worse and more unbearable. After consulting with nurses, Dr. Nigam finally verifies that they will order her another drug.

Hours pass, and Pam's vitals stabilize. Aides wheel her to her own hospital room.

"I'm right here with you," Jody keeps assuring Pam. "It'll be OK."

Pam's face scrunches in pain as she moves her head slightly to the side.

"Pam they're getting you something," Jody says. "Try to stay focused. The surgery went really well."

Jody leans beside her sister's bed, positions her arm on the bar on the bed and lays her head on her arm while she watches Pam. Jody has been by her side more than a year now, ever since Pam called to say she found a lump. Today, Jody continues to be there for Pam as she comforts her while they wait for more drugs from the doctor. Jody has already planned to stay the night at the hospital and sleep in the chair that reclines into a bed. She knows this chair quite well; she slept in a similar one for several days after Pam's 12-hour surgery last January.

"We think we got all the disease," Dr. Nigam said to Jody and Lambros in the waiting room. During Pam's first visit with Dr. Nigam, he said the best-case scenario would be to cure her with this procedure. This is the hope getting all of them through the pains of post-surgery.

For a second, Pam struggles to open her eyes. Her surgical cap is gone. She is out of surgery, and she has survived.

From her hospital bed, she looks out, briefly, as if awakening to a more beautiful world, and forms a hint of a smile. It is over.

Two days later, Pam, in her silk floral pajamas, sits up slowly so as not to move the lower part of her torso. Still in the hospital, she's in danger of liver failure. In front of her is a tray consisting of a plate of picked-at grapes and cottage cheese, which is the first meal she's managed to eat since her couple bits of turkey at Jody's house. And even though Halloween is over, she finally gets her chocolate, as a piece of chocolate cake accompanies her food.

Pam and Jody are still together as they watch TV in Pam's hospital room. Jody will not leave Pam's side unless someone is there to take over.

This is the worst pain she's ever experienced, Pam says, worse than the bilateral mastectomy and breast reconstruction. She hasn't even been fully coherent until that morning. They are keeping her in the hospital until her enzymes become close to normal in her liver. She is experiencing what one might endure with a severe case of Hepatitis C, which attacks the liver. After three weeks of recovery in and out of the hospital, she will learn that the surgery worked, and she will be in remission.

At that moment, though, she feels well enough to raise her bed so she can sit up.

Pam's bed readjusts to her elevated position by filling up with air, and the pump's motors make a loud noise. The rumble sounds like an airplane picking up its landing gear and shifting its wings for flight.

"It sounds like an airplane taking off," Pam jokes as her bed inflates automatically.

"She's taking off," Jody laughs.

"Don't make me laugh," Pam says to Jody. It hurts her to laugh.

The bed continues making its airplane sound.

"Prepare for liftoff," Jody says.

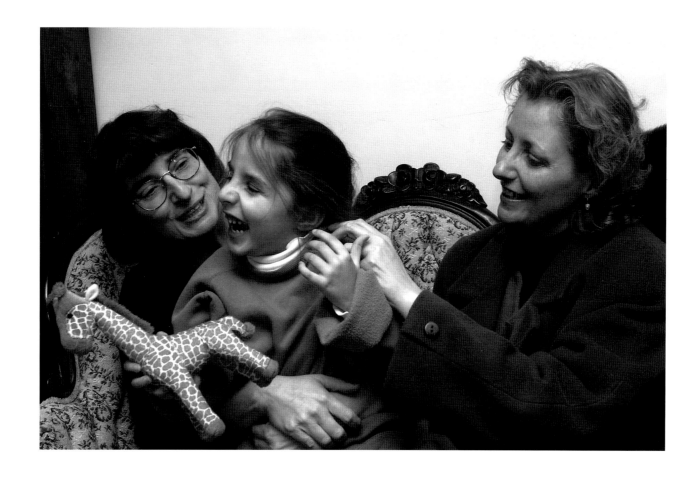

The legacy of cancer haunts Jody, Joey, and Pam, but it has brought them closer as well.

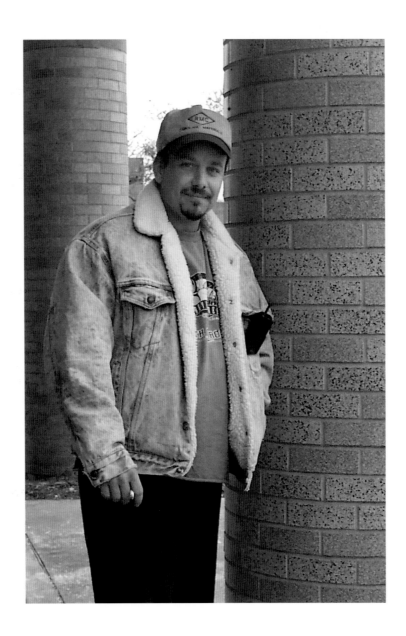

VERNON M. KNODE III

text by EUNICE ROHRER

The nurse fastens a black tourniquet with a buckle around Vernon Knode's bulging right bicep and pulls it tight. She cleans the underside of his elbow with a square white swatch of material presoaked with antiseptic and picks up a three-inch long needle with a syringe.

Junior had been leaning back, resting against his dad's shoulder, but sits forward and watches with fascination when the needle appears. Vernon glances down at his son, then up and away as the needle slides smoothly into his arm. Little Junior stares straight at the bulging vein—oversized Uno cards clutched tightly in his hands but game forgotten. He glances worriedly up at the nurse once and continues to take in every detail as she loosens the tourniquet and switches vials to get two test tube samples of Vernon's blood.

Vernon laughs nervously as he watches his son's reaction. The nurse completes the blood draw, placing a cotton ball on the spot and indicating to Vernon to apply pressure. Vernon covers the cotton ball tightly with his left hand. With his right he nudges Junior's shoulder and asks, "You want one of them? It don't hurt."

Junior shrugs his shoulders and uses the Uno cards to brush his long hair out of his eyes.

Vernon M. Knode takes a break outside the Mary Babb Randolph Cancer Center before his three-hour drive home. In February 2001, he was diagnosed with chronic mylogenous leukemia, inheriting a family legacy of cancer. Until recently, those afflicted with CML—one of the rarest, yet mildest forms of leukemia—had a 32 percent chance of remission, but new drugs offer a glimmer of hope.

photographs by EUNICE ROHRER

His father repeats, "You want a needle?" This time Junior shakes his head no and begins to smile faintly again.

The nurse places tape over the area, and father and son watch seriously, their heads close together. As she cleans the treatment area, Vernon shifts Junior to the other side of his lap. Junior is smiling again and lifts the cards up for his dad to play with him.

———

Junior is only about three feet tall, but he has big, dark eyes and straight brown hair that falls freely four inches past the collar of his yellow shirt, which is too large for him. Earlier today, as they walked through the lobby of the Mary Babb Randolph Cancer Center, he tried to shrug out of his jacket with one arm, while tugging at his dad's hand with the other.

When they enter the exam room, he hops up onto the bed beside his dad, crinkling the paper sheet. Junior still wants to play Uno. Vernon shuffles out the cards with Winnie the Pooh on the back of them, and an impromptu game begins. It is as if they are struggling for some scrap of normalcy in the sterile surroundings.

They laugh, tease and slap cards while waiting for the doctors to come perform a bone marrow aspiration. The results will determine whether Vernon is going into remission from chronic mylogenic leukemia.

"Uno!" Vernon calls.

"Huh uh!" Junior protests.

"I only got one card left," Vernon explains gently to Junior, waving the Uno card.

Vernon has been taking Gleevec, a chemotherapy pill, for more than 10 months. He should be showing signs of improvement at the chromosomal level by now. Regular biopsies will tell whether Vernon is on the path to regaining his health. The hope is that the biopsies will reveal a larger number of normal cells than abnormal cells in Vernon's bone marrow. If this is maintained for five years or more, he will be in remission. Currently, 32 percent of chronic mylogenous leukemia, or CML, patients have a chance of remission, but that statistic was calculated before some of the newer drugs were available.

—·—

He is just 33 years old, but Vernon Marcellous Knode III has already inherited much from his family: his father and grandfather's name, a heritage of hard work, and a family legacy of cancer.

All four of Vernon's grandparents died from different forms of cancer. Many of his aunts and uncles and even cousins have died of cancer or currently have it. Finally, two of Vernon's nieces have had cancer and his sister, Kim, was diagnosed with cancer in October 2002. Vernon intends to fight his condition, and with the support of his mother and other family members, he is focused on changing a family legacy. He actively seeks medical help now, unlike his father, who is now deceased.

Vernon Sr. was a diesel mechanic and equipment operator, who also did excavating for a living. He passed his love of heavy equipment on to his son. Vernon III has operated loaders, bull-dozers, and tractor-trailers over the years.

When Vernon was 26, his father succumbed to throat and lung cancer, exacerbated by years of heavy drinking. Vernon Knode Sr. was only 52 at the time of his death. Vernon Sr. disliked going to doctors and put it off until "he got to the point where he just couldn't take it," the younger Vernon says.

Vernon Sr. went to the VA center, and they gave him 30 days to live. They said he had throat cancer. Vernon had moved to North Carolina by that time but returned to visit his father.

"He told me not to come back again, so I didn't come back. Sometimes, it's better to remember somebody looking at you," Vernon says.

—·—

Vernon was handed his legacy almost from the moment of his birth—when he received the family name. Vernon Marcellous Knode III was born March 6, 1970, at Washington County Hospital in Hagerstown, Maryland. His parents, Virginia and Vernon Knode Sr., named their son after his father and grandfather, both of whom were committed to lives of hard work in

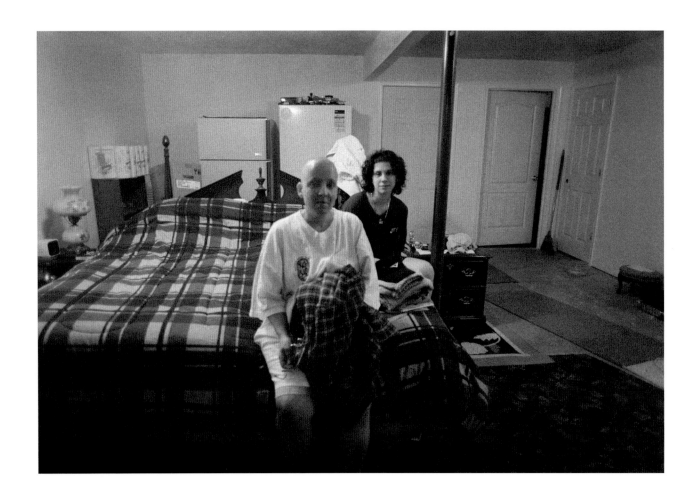

Vernon's sister Kim and niece Jessica (his sister Angie's daughter), take a break from cleaning up the basement bedroom at his mother's home in Martinsburg, West Virginia. Once a heavy equipment operator, Vernon quit his job and moved back from North Carolina when he became ill. Now in remission, Vernon goes to a job in North Carolina for weeks at a time. Vernon isn't supposed to be working, but with no insurance to cover his treatments, he has no alternative.

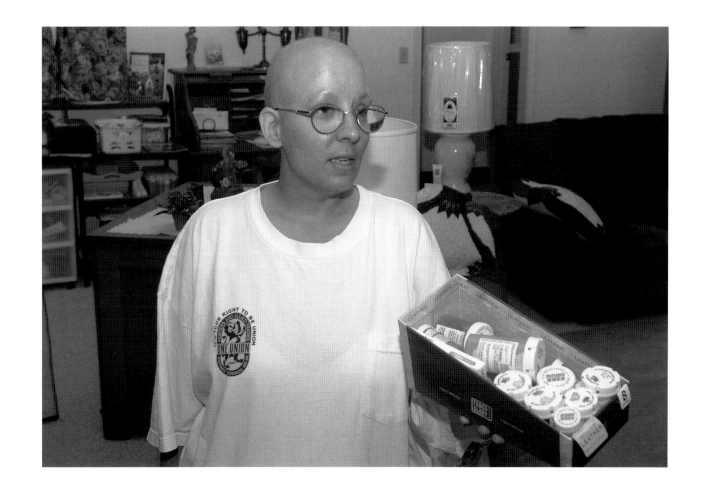

Vernon's sister Kim currently lives with her mother in Martinsburg while struggling with her own cancer. Kim is one of seven members of Vernon's family to have battled cancer. She has undergone extensive chemotherapy and surgery.

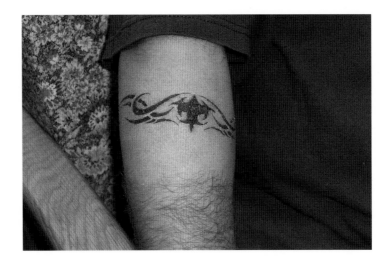

construction or heavy machinery operation. Virginia has married Jack Henratta since Vernon Sr.'s death.

Vernon's sisters are Angela VanMetre and Kimberly Nett, both a few years older than he is. When Kim was small, she wanted to nickname her little brother Butch, but she couldn't pronounce it right so she had to settle for something simpler.

Every weekend, the children watched Yogi Bear and his little sidekick Boo Boo, and that was where he got his nickname, Boo Boo. To this day, Vernon's mother and sisters call him Boo.

In 1975, Virginia moved the children to Martinsburg, West Virginia. Vernon Sr. had left the family by then. These were not easy times for the children or Virginia, who worked at night carving keys and pull knobs for large church organs to provide for her family.

Vernon's mother says he was a "good little kid … just a typical little boy." He always had long hair when he was younger.

Vernon got his first tattoo, a swastika, at age 15. After an orthopedic resident—a middle-aged Jewish man—became upset, Vernon had it inked over into a new design. When asked why he originally chose a swastika, he replied, "Just young and dumb."

When he was a small child, Vernon came down with something like pneumonia every winter. He had to be hospitalized and put in an oxygen tent. His doctors said he would outgrow it, and he did, but not before he lost his hearing in one ear due to infection. Regardless of his experiences with illness in his youth, Vernon was already following in his father's footsteps.

"My idea of being a kid was being with my dad. Whatever he was doing, that's what I wanted to do," Vernon said. He would go to whatever job site his dad was currently working on.

As a child, Vernon went to Boonsboro Elementary and North Middle School. Later, he attended Martinsburg High School. He started listening to heavy metal music—his favorite was Metallica, but he liked Led Zeppelin and KISS, too. Other habits of Vernon's changed about this time as well. When he was younger, Vernon went to church every Sunday, but when he was 12 or 13 he quit going.

"I kinda went the opposite direction," Vernon recalled.

He was only 15 when he took the car his father gave him and left home to strike out on his own because he didn't want to cause hard feelings in the family. His mother remembers it this way: "Boo didn't want to live with me and he didn't want to live with his daddy because he didn't want either of us to think he was taking sides."

During his later teenage years, Vernon lived with his sister, Kim. She says her little brother has always liked to follow her wherever she goes.

"I woke up one morning from him knocking on my door. There he was with his Jeep and motorcycle and all he owned," Kim said. She kept an eye out for Vernon and helped him get a job working for Bill Magnum, nicknamed Monkey, who owned Magnum Concrete near High Point, North Carolina.

The crews usually worked 12 to 15 hours a day. In the winter, a typical workday might be even longer because the concrete took more time to set. Vernon always worked the longest because he set the forms for the next day's job before leaving in the evening.

After he arrived home at night, Vernon liked to work on the pickup trucks or race cars.

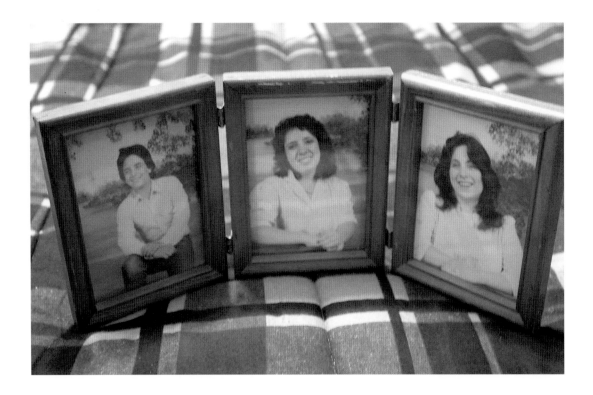

He listened to heavy metal while he "threw some wrenches around," as he calls it. Kim remembered he always stayed busy, and he played father figure to her kids. He took them to truck races.

During those years, Vernon lived by himself in a company house his employer provided. Kim later moved out west to California for a while when her brother was busy with work and his own small family.

The owner of the company and their boss, Bill Magnum, said he first met Vernon about 12 years ago.

A legacy of cancer haunts Vernon's family. From left to right: Vernon at 14, Kim at 16, and Angie at 17. Their father, all four of their grandparents along with several aunts, uncles and cousins have died from different forms of cancer. Two nieces currently have cancer; Vernon was diagnosed with cancer in 2001 and Kim in 2002. Of the three siblings, only Angie is cancer-free.

"I raised that boy," Magnum said. "He was good to me." Vernon's boss describes him this way, "About like everybody else at 18, wild."

———

Then in 1998, his girlfriend got pregnant. Their son, Vernon Marcellous Knode IV, was born on March 10, 1999. As the baby grew, a neighbor next door, Ruth O'Sullivan, took an interest in him and often babysat.

"Oh, I loved that baby," she said. "I got him a plastic wheelbarrow one time. If you could have seen that child's face! He loved his Mamaw. The other neighbors used to say, 'There goes Miss Ruthie with her baby'," Ruth chuckled.

"Good little boy. Looks like Vernon," Magnum remembers of the smallest Vernon. To avoid confusion, they began calling the boy Junior.

His son wanted to do whatever Vernon did around the house.

"Ever since the day he started walking, he'd be out there up underneath the car with me," Vernon said. If Vernon got a shovel, Junior had to have a shovel. So they would plant flowers together. "I'd dig and he'd plant and water," Vernon remembers.

Before Junior was born, Vernon had a "don't care" attitude toward life. He says he wouldn't have cared if someone shot him. Since he has a son, he says he has something to live for now.

Bill Magnum, Vernon's employer for more than a decade, had noticed a change in Vernon's energy level soon after his son was born. Magnum said you could tell he was sick. While Vernon may not have known he was seriously ill, he must have been aware that something was not right.

Even his oldest sister, Angie, who now lived in the apartment upstairs, tried to get him to find out what was wrong. Angie kept hearing him gagging—she could hear everything from his apartment. She kept telling him, "Boo, something's wrong." However, much like their father, Vernon refused to go to a doctor. He kept telling Angie nothing was wrong.

———

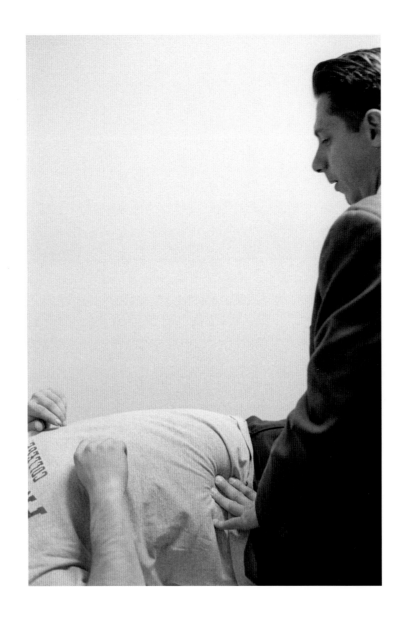

*Vernon's illness has encompassed more than cancer. He has regular
check ups with Dr. Biundo, an orthopedic doctor.*

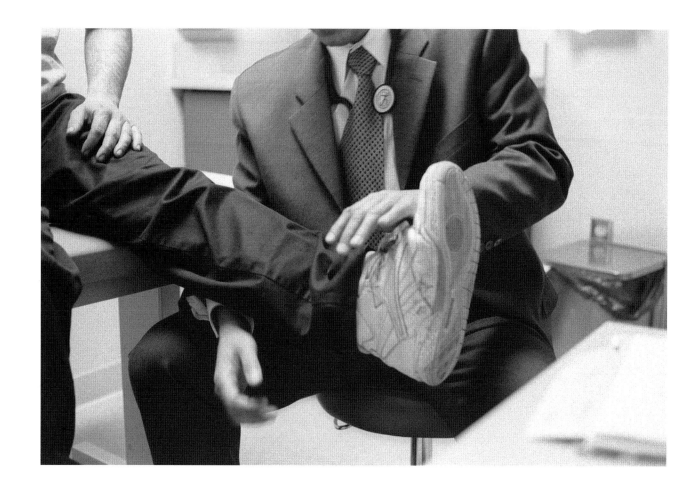

Vernon's 12-hour workdays as a heavy equipment operator have led to chronic muscle and joint pain as well as back pain and numbness in his legs and feet.

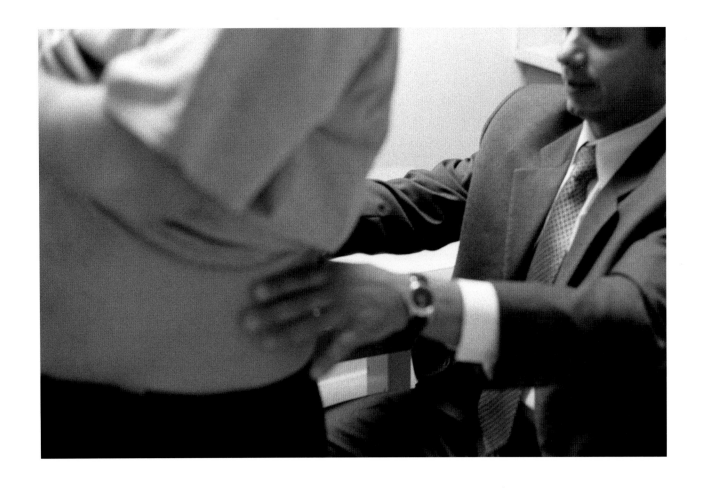

Doctors fear that part of Vernon's joint and nerve problems are a result of working long hours throughout his illness. Although Dr. Biundo feels it is probably osteoarthritis, it could be symptoms of CML leukemia.

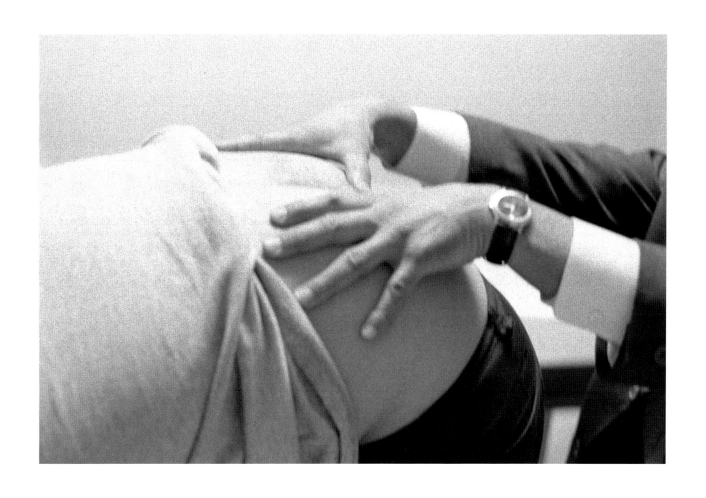

Vernon planned to get a five-year renewal for his driver's license on February 14, 2001. But that Valentine's Day did not turn out as he expected.

Rain pelted down as Vernon drove the beige and white 1986 Chevrolet pickup he'd nicknamed Dully to the Department of Motor Vehicles station near High Point, North Carolina. He'd bought a heavy-duty pickup because his work-oriented life did not justify a car.

First, Vernon paid his fees and took the written test. Then the vision test proved to be more difficult for Vernon than it should have been. Vernon had realized for some time that he had a hole in the middle of his frontal vision, so he went straight to a little eye center in High Point to see what was actually wrong.

After a thorough exam, which found hemorrhaging in the back of his eye, followed by blood work at a lab, Vernon was sent home.

———

At eight a.m. the next day, he received a call from the doctor, who told Vernon he needed to come to the office right away. His white blood cell count was 365,000. Normally, white blood cell counts run between 5,000 and 10,000. If it had gone much higher, he could have just collapsed.

Vernon was told he probably had CML, a cancer of the blood. The date was February 15, 2001. He was ordered to go home, get packed and check in as a patient at 2 p.m. They had a room waiting for him at Baptist Hospital.

———

As soon as he heard this news, Vernon told Bill Magnum he wouldn't be coming to work that day, maybe never.

"I called him very first thing. Me and him was real close, you know. He was like my daddy," Vernon says.

He also called his sister, Angie, to let her and his family know what was happening. Then Vernon left for the hospital but didn't drive directly there. He stopped along the way at Five Point Motors. From there he called a couple of people he was doing jobs for, just to let them know what was going on and that he was not going to be around for awhile. He wanted to settle his affairs because he didn't know how long he would be gone.

———

Soon after she received the message that her son was ill, Vernon's mother, Virginia Henratta, drove from her home in Martinsburg to the hospital in North Carolina. Virginia needed to see Vernon for herself, arriving while he was still in the hospital.

"When I first got there he was taking it OK," Virginia said. From the first day she learned about her son's condition, Virginia tried to convince him to move home with her.

In July 2001, five months after he was diagnosed, Vernon's sister, Kim, just showed up at Vernon's place. She had been living in San Diego, California, but had a disturbing dream that someone in the family was sick, says Virginia.

"She thought it was me," Virginia said. Kim was shocked to hear the news about her younger brother. The two of them had not kept in touch well in recent years, but had retained a bond since childhood.

———

After he was admitted, Vernon remained in the hospital on an intravenous drip bag for the next four days. He was given fluids and started on Hydrea pills immediately. His white cell counts were stabilized enough for him to leave the hospital and return to his home in North Carolina within four days. He began regular visits to Wake Forest Medical Center.

His doctors at Wake Forest told Vernon that he would probably need a bone-marrow transplant in six months. The primary goal for them was to control his white blood cell count. If they couldn't control his white cell level, that was when he was supposed to start worrying. But the only thing they told Vernon to do was to expect the best but prepare for the worst.

After that Vernon had to go see a doctor every week. He tried not to let the medical appointments interfere with his plans for the day. If he had an appointment at 2 p.m., he would work until 1 or 1:30 p.m.. He says he was usually late, but if he arrived by 4 p.m. the medical staff was happy. He only wanted them to check his white cell count, and then he was back at the job site again.

"I'd usually take the dump truck or anything, as long as it would fit up in the parking deck," Vernon recalled with a grin.

In 2001, Vernon moved back home to Martinsburg to live with his mother, and he became a patient at the Mary Babb Randolph Cancer Center. During one part of the move, Vernon's mother was driving a tractor-trailer full of Vernon's possessions on the interstate when it started to jackknife. "I just put on the brakes and rode it out," Virginia said.

This also seems to be her approach to caring for Vernon. Virginia says she must be the strong one in the family, or she wouldn't be given so much trouble to endure in her life. Helping with the physical part of moving items from North Carolina to her home was only one aspect of having her son come back to stay with her, however.

It had been approximately 17 years since the two of them had shared living space together.

"It's not that often you have your 30-something son come back home to live with you," Virginia said as she sat quietly in the waiting room of the Cancer Center in Morgantown. As she continued to stitch on a colorful green and rose quilt patch, Virginia said she planned to be there to support her son throughout his treatment.

"He's my only son and the baby," she said.

It is Valentine's Day 2002, one year after Vernon's diagnosis and he is visiting the Cancer Center in Morgantown with his mother along to help on the three-hour drive home.

"Your counts are totally normal," says Marcel Devetten, MD, during Vernon's regular visit to the Cancer Center. Vernon has had a positive hematological response since he began taking four Gleevec pills a day. His blood counts are as normal as a perfectly healthy individual's, but not his chromosomes.

"We'll stick to our original plan," Dr. Devetten continues. "Do a bone-marrow [biopsy] on the Gleevec in probably about three months and look at the chromosome studies at that time."

"Now the Gleevec should get rid of the blasts [immature white blood cells] in my marrow?" Vernon asks.

"Yes, it should," Dr. Devetten says. "But that's what we will have to check, of course, in a couple months."

"Then even if the blasts go out, I still have to take it?"

"Yeah, if it works. The idea is people are pretty much on it indefinitely. If it's going to stop, then it will not be until maybe five or 10 years from now."

Until then, Vernon will have bone marrow biopsies every few months to check the status of his disease at the chromosomal level. His next biopsy takes place on May 2, 2002.

———

When he arrives for his first bone marrow biopsy at the Cancer Center, Vernon has a blood sample drawn, as usual, to determine the white cell count in his blood.

When the surgical technicians enter the room to prepare Vernon for surgery, he climbs up and lies face down on the exam table.

John Rizzo, the physician's assistant who will be doing the bone marrow biopsy today, pulls the khakis down almost to Vernon's buttocks and swabs the lower back and upper buttocks area with an orange Betadine solution three times. Rizzo places a blue paper sheet with a square hole in the middle of it over the area and unwraps a lab kit. He selects a four-inch needle and a vial of two percent Lanocaine to numb the tissue around the hip bone. Next, Rizzo picks up a six-inch, blue-handled instrument from the cart and sticks it gently into the numbed tissue until it is near the bone. He begins to turn it with more pressure and a twisting motion of his hand.

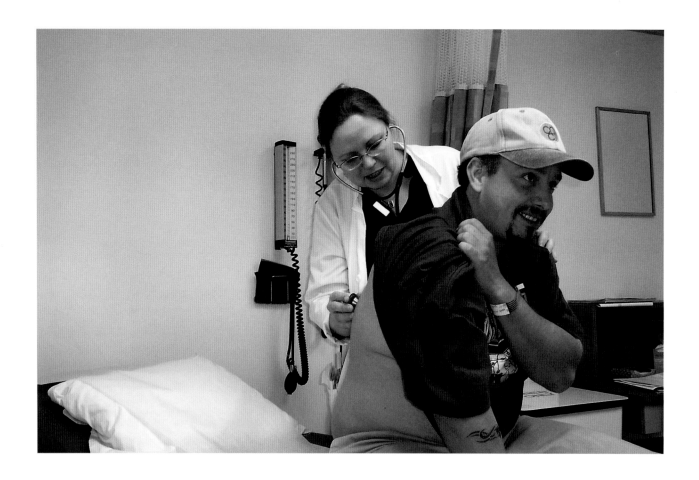

Vernon's new physicians, Dr. Schunn and Dr. Erickson, explain his treatment options to him (above right). Vernon spends much of the appointment joking about having a bone marrow transplant, and while it is not his first option, he requests to remain in the donor list database. At a routine appointment, Dr. Schunn checks the condition of his lungs (above).

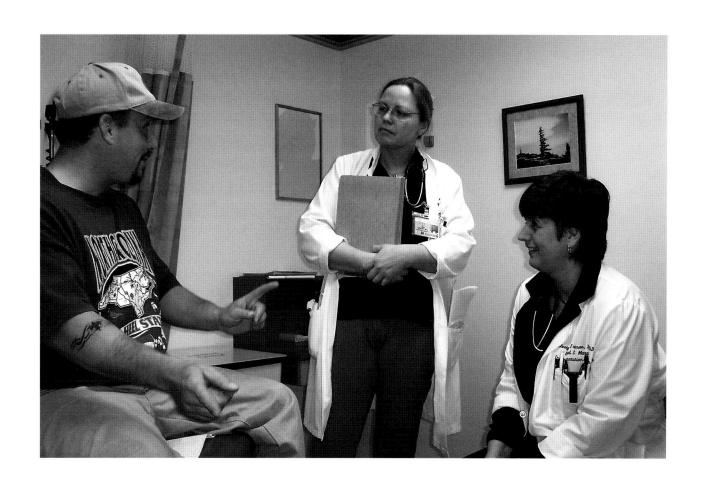

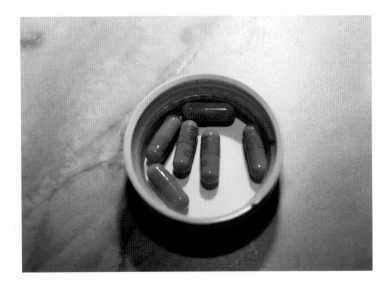

Within 30 seconds he is satisfied that it is in place. He flips out a movable section in the top of the handle and replaces it with a syringe. There is a hollow needle already inside the instrument where the syringe attaches.

"All right, I'm getting ready to pull it out—that pressure feeling. So try to hold still, and we'll do it real quick here," Rizzo says. He pumps on the syringe three times to get enough bone marrow fluid and hands the red liquid to Joyce Vincent, the laboratory technician.

Vincent squirts the bone marrow fluid into three vials, one each with red, yellow and lavender stopper caps. She shakes the vials and places them in a yellow crate. Next Vincent puts several drops on a slanting clear plate, the size and shape of a small ruler, where the liquid runs down and soaks into a paper towel.

She picks up small, clear slide plates and wipes some of the fluid onto each one, topping the

For Vernon, Gleevec is a miracle drug. Coming on the market at the moment when Vernon was diagnosed with cancer, Gleevec provided an alternative to a bone marrow transplant. Vernon was not eligible to receive the experimental drug while in North Carolina, so he moved to West Virginia to begin treatment. The company mails the pills to him as part of a patient program.

plates with another one of identical size. Vincent turns one plate toward the light to check if she is getting enough spicules—bone cells. The cells are visible to the naked eye and can be seen on each slide. The purpose is to allow the slides to stain and dry so she can look at them through a microscope later.

Rizzo removes the blue-handled instrument and holds a swab with pressure on the spot for a few seconds to stop the bleeding. Then he gathers the used swabs, empty packaging and crumples the paper sheet, tossing them into the red biohazard box. The lab will have the results back in a week.

This is not Vernon's first biopsy and by now he knows the drill. He will be sore in his right leg for two weeks. He gets off the exam bed, tucks his shirt in and hurries outside for a cigarette.

———

A week later Vernon was working on the neighbor's farm between rainstorms when the lab results became available. He had not tried calling to learn what the lab results were yet because he "didn't really want to know." Instead, he waited and waited until his next appointment on June 20, six weeks after the biopsy, to hear how it turned out.

He did talk to someone from the Cancer Center about potential matches in the meantime. They asked if he wanted to keep his donor matches current in the database, and he said they could. "I was worried," Vernon said, admitting fear for the first time since January 2002.

———

At Vernon's next visit to the Cancer Center, Dr. Devetten had his biopsy results ready to discuss with him. The test results, from 20 chromosomes, came back with four healthy chromosomes and 16 abnormal chromosomes. Dr. Devetten was hoping the abnormal count would go down to seven or eight. Dr. Devetten said this doesn't mean the Gleevec won't eventually work, but that the treatment needs to continue. Bone marrow biopsies need to be continued every couple months or so.

Dr. Devetten says the Gleevec is helping, but not quite as much as he hoped. Before any treatment, Vernon had 20 out of 20 abnormal chromosomes.

Vernon had to struggle with the realization that he might need to slow down and take life easier. He had been so independent all his life.

Nevertheless, Vernon is the type of person who needs to stay busy, so when he first moved into his mom's house, he helped out a neighbor man on a nearby farm. Vernon used to live for work and a paycheck. He says he was always buying things. Now he is trying to find life in a different state, with a different family, and through a new drug, Gleevec.

———

Vernon has been making some lifestyle changes besides the physical move home to his mother's place. He cut back on the beers and quit drinking caffeine altogether. A local physician discovered acid reflux had caused the gagging, and caffeine worsens that condition. He tried to quit smoking, but in order to get the patch he would have had to sit through some classes, and the bother wasn't worth it, according to him.

In Vernon's room in his mother's house, a pack of Basic Ultralights and a Coors Light bottle sit empty on the nightstand to the left of the four-poster bed.

There is a Sanyo 17-inch TV across from the bed and a foam cheering hand above the bed. On the dresser a certificate of baptism states that Vernon Marcellous Knode III was christened on March 29, 1970, at the Holy Trinity Lutheran Church when he was 23 days old.

Also on the dresser are a stack of CDs including Nirvana and Sting. A Mary Chapin Carpenter CD is still in the wrapper. A real coonskin cap hangs from the mirror.

———

It is late summertime, and Vernon has been doing outside work at his mom's house in Martinsburg and working for a landscaping company called Greenside Up.

His job involves trimming bushes and cutting trees down. He uses the chain saw and skid loader to clear brush in a backyard not far from Virginia's.

At the site where he is clearing the area of trees and brush, Vernon jumps down from the red cab of the dump truck and heads for the machine he spends most of his time in these days. It is a black and yellow New Holland LX 465 skid loader with the bucket on it. Vernon calls it a Bobcat. He can manipulate the hand controls with dexterity, but lately he's been getting some numbness in his hands.

Vernon works steadily, a cigarette dangling from his mouth the whole time. The machete swiftly tears the branches from the pine tree to be crushed under the bucket of the loader. The smaller brush he drags together in a pile with the bucket, then scoops it repeatedly into the bed of the dump truck.

The engine whines as he swivels and bounces on the machine, occasionally pulling the loader onto its back two wheels with the bucket raised overhead. Engine exhaust and the scent of fresh pine fill the air.

When the dump truck is full, Vernon switches off the loader, takes a real smoke break, and then climbs back into the 1979 F-700 Ford dump truck to haul the brush away. After a meandering drive back to the Henrattas', he empties the truck in the woods behind the house.

In October 2002, Vernon learned that his sister, Kim, has cancer. She had a major operation, which removed large tumors from her abdomen. He says he wasn't surprised by the news.

"In our family, it's a surprise if you don't have cancer," Vernon says.

Kim has moved to Martinsburg to live at the Henratta home with her mother, Virginia, and stepdad, Jack. She is on chemo treatments and is doing OK. Vernon stays there, too, when he isn't doing construction work in North Carolina. However, he let Kim have his bedroom right off the family room upstairs. He now has a room in the basement.

Also, in October 2002, two days before Halloween, Vernon drove to Tennessee to see his son, Junior. Daisy, his ex-girlfriend, let him stay a few days and then bring Junior back to Martinsburg until November 24, allowing Vernon to spend almost a month with his son. Junior insists on going everywhere with his dad, including visits to the Cancer Center.

As Vernon waits to leave the exam room, the registered nurse who works for Dr. Devetten walks in.

"That your son?" the nurse asks.

"Yeah," Vernon says.

"He looks like you," the nurse says, handing Vernon his white cell counts, which are normal again.

"When I come up Monday, is there anything I can do for him?" Vernon asks, indicating Junior. He would like his son to be checked for cancer because of the increasingly early onset of cancer in his family. Vernon's grandfather, Vernon I, was diagnosed with cancer in his 70s, Vernon Sr. in his 50s and now Vernon III in his 30s. But they all had different forms of the disease.

"It's dropping [every] 20 years. Now there's one in her teens [Vernon's niece who is in remission]." Dr. Devetten says the type of leukemia Vernon has is not hereditary. Vernon doesn't quite believe this.

"The main thing is catching it early," Ryan adds. "Just go see a doctor."

Junior, now in his father's arms, looks up at his dad and makes a funny face. Everyone laughs.

When they reach the lobby, Vernon puts Junior down to play. He has to wait in line several minutes to schedule his next appointment.

Meanwhile, Junior plays with the electric doors and waves to strangers. Finally, his appointment made, Vernon holds his son's hand as they walk out the doors and away from the Cancer Center.

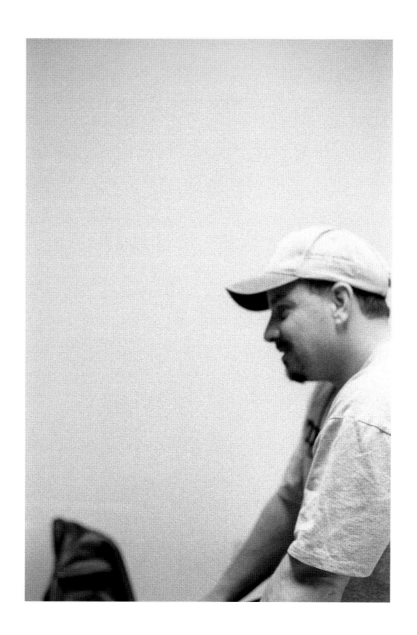

Vernon used to live for work and a paycheck. He says he was always buying things. Now he is trying to find life in a different state, with a different family, and through a new treatment.

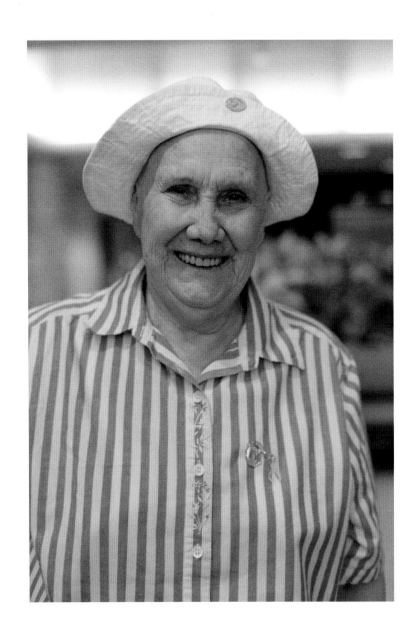

BANANA BREAD

text by JAN LAUREN BOYLES

DECEMBER 2002

Within the labyrinthine corridors of the Mary Babb Randolph Cancer Center lies a space—no larger than a broom closet—that serves as the nerve center for John Rogers, MD, and his team. Dr. Rogers, Nurse Practitioner Vidya Brown, and a pair of registered nurses begin this morning there, huddle d over a calculator. While punching the numbers to determine proper doses of chemotherapy, the teammates listen to Dr. Rogers as if he were a starting quarterback giving directions for the next play, or in this case—the next treatment option. But in their branch of medicine, every option is a "Hail Mary" play.

According to the numbers, the mass within this patient's chest has decreased significantly. In response to the good news, Dr. Rogers discreetly smiles and takes a tiny sip from a cup of ice water; its liquid has gathered condensation on the files scattered upon his desk. Dr. Rogers savors the small victories, whatever their form.

On this morning, Dr. Rogers will see 13 patients.

Brown presents Dr. Rogers with a synopsis of each patient's history with the

---

Geraldine Thomas was diagnosed in 2001 with advanced lung cancer. Although confronted with a terminal illness, Geraldine's gregarious nature and joyous spirit sustained not only herself but the doctors and nurses whose job it was to treat her. Nurse Practitioner Vidya Brown recalls the first time the two met: "I won't give you a handshake, honey, I only give hugs," Geraldine promised.

photographs by BARBARA GRIFFIN

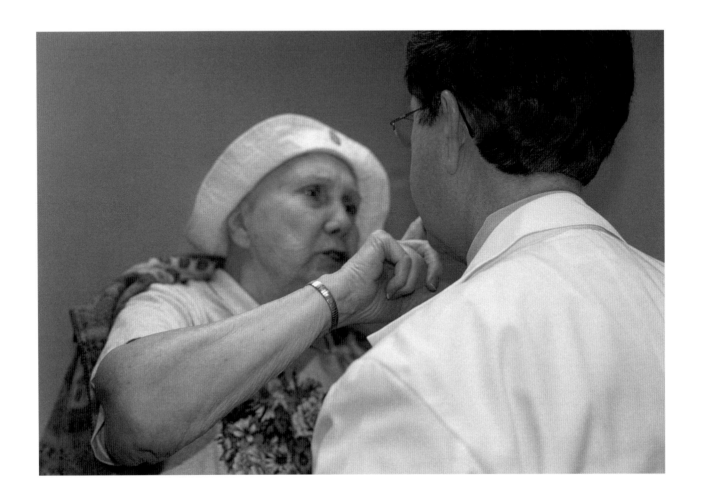

Geraldine brings freshly baked banana bread from her home in Summersville, West Virginia, to each doctor's appointment, chemotherapy or radiation session. In a playful gesture, she wipes the remaining crumbs from Dr. Rogers' face.

disease, current treatment pattern and related symptoms. Subsequently, the pair confer about what path will be best applicable to each patient.

One such patient, Geraldine Thomas, was diagnosed with lung cancer in 2001. She had been coughing up large quantities of blood nightly. She first dismissed it as a broken blood vessel. But Geraldine's son, Dana, believed that her episodes indicated a greater health concern, especially after he found a wastebasket full of Kleenex and blood at her home.

Geraldine suffers from locally advanced lung cancer. Initially, this diagnosis confirmed that the cancer was confined to a single organ of the body and had not yet spread to the bloodstream.

"When the doctor said 'You got cancer,' it was just a relief to know that he found something, you know," Thomas said. "So I just go with the flow, that's what I say to 'em. I just go with the flow."

———

Clad in a striped blue shirt, solid red tie, khakis and lab coat, Dr. Rogers gingerly knocks on the door of examining room eight for another meeting with Geraldine. While Dr. Rogers may appear distant and quiet to spectators, the oncologist developed an immediate connection with the gregarious Geraldine. "I remember the first time that I met Geraldine," Dr. Rogers said. "I thought that instantly she was a strong and delightful woman."

Vidya Brown also clearly recollects the first time she entered Geraldine's examining room. She remembers kindly extending her delicate hand to the 75-year-old as means of introduction. Geraldine, however, had other ideas.

"I remember the very first words Geraldine told me," Brown said. "She vowed to me, 'I won't give you a handshake, honey, I only give hugs,' " Brown parodied in her best replication of a southern West Virginian accent, albeit with overt New England intonation.

"After that encounter with Geraldine, I remember thinking, not only is this woman amazing, but she is a downright inspiration," Brown said.

———

On this morning, Geraldine's blue eyes are shadowed by an oversized white bucket hat with an enormous brim. The only feature visible from this angle is her smile. She wears the cap to shield her newly bald head, and she wears the grin as a delicate disguise to the observer.

Every trip to West Virginia University's Mary Babb Randolph Cancer Center takes approximately two hours driving time from Geraldine's home in Summersville, West Virginia. She is always accompanied by a member of the family, whether it be her sister, Mary, or son, Dana. For early morning appointments, Geraldine arrives the night before and sleeps overnight in the Cancer Center's Family House—a set of hotel-like suites for patients and their families.

This morning, with fragile hands, Geraldine struggles to reach a mound of crumpled aluminum foil lying on a nearby counter. She unwraps the package with precision, painstakingly unfolding each crease of the outer paper.

"Would y'all care for a piece of banana bread?" Geraldine Thomas asks Dr. Rogers and Brown in her cozy accent. "It's tradition, ya know."

She passes the foil's contents to the observers seated on mismatched stools lining the stark, white walls of the examining room. Everyone takes a slice and eats it with a smile. Geraldine brings the fresh banana bread from her home to each chemotherapy and radiation session.

"She never forgets it. Never," Brown says, grinning. "When she comes with her banana bread, it's the highlight of my day."

While personable with each patient, Dr. Rogers' protocol of questions is routine. In his barely legible handwriting, he scrawls symptoms pertaining to appetite, energy and level of activity in her file.

However procedural his initial exchange, Dr. Rogers develops special ways of speaking with each patient. The average duration of Dr. Rogers' consultations is 15 minutes, with plenty of time for questions and answers. But consultations with Geraldine tend to last a bit longer.

"There's always a balance between reading charts and spending time," Dr. Rogers said. "Even though I want to do my homework in here before I visit the patients, I want to spend as much time with the people as humanly possible, to talk to them face to face."

But not every appointment is mechanical, according to Dr. Rogers.

Dr. Rogers' everyday duties include relating heartbreaking, life-changing information to his patients, a process with which the oncologist is all too familiar. But imparting that moment of truth—a diagnosis, setback or remission in the fight against cancer—has not become easier as the years have passed.

In Geraldine's case, further testing ruled out surgery because Geraldine's tumor was located in the lower right quadrant of the lung, making it impossible to operate. Due to the radiation therapy, the tumor initially shrank 50 percent. However, during summer 2002, the tumor began growing again, becoming even larger than before.

Dr. Rogers vividly recalls when he had to tell Geraldine.

"I always try to be truthful," Dr. Rogers said as a single tear streamed down his face. "I never want to keep information from them. In other words, I don't try to back up a truck and dump bad news on people. I try to inform my patients in a gentle but truthful way."

Dr. Rogers admits that it never gets any easier to speak frankly about his patients' mortality. In the majority of cases, the oncologist is aware how much time each patient has to live. Dr. Rogers wasn't sure in Geraldine's case.

"But I've learned the importance of not letting time slide—of getting to know someone and receiving more from them," Dr. Rogers said.

"I think that patients appreciate Dr. Rogers' straightforward approach," Brown said. "While some patients may want their news a little more sugar-coated, I respect Dr. Rogers for telling the truth to his patients. He's extremely empathetic and sensitive. Dr. Rogers truly wants to make a difference. I think that as a result, patients would rather see their physician as strong and invincible than weak and vulnerable. He's their fighter."

His gentle yet "fighting" demeanor has emerged from 27 years of advising patients like Geraldine. The oncologist has spent his entire career in West Virginia.

As part of their hectic schedule, Dr. Rogers and Brown shuttle between appointments to another larger office in a separate wing of the center. Among numerous cubicle work-spaces, two vertically-positioned, black-and-white computer screens allow the oncologist to view

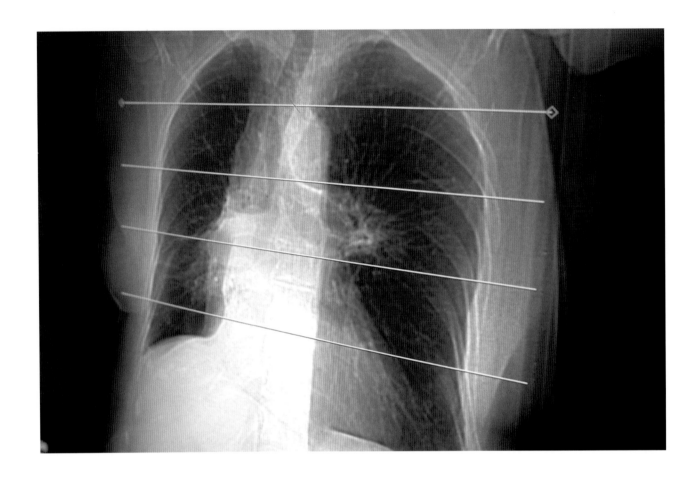

At the Mary Babb Randolph Cancer Center, Geraldine undergoes daily radiation therapy for six weeks with the hope of shrinking the inoperable tumor. Initially, the radiation treatments seem to succeed in reducing its size. Months later, Geraldine's scan shows a growing tumor and the early signs of pneumonia that will eventually bring a halt to treatments.

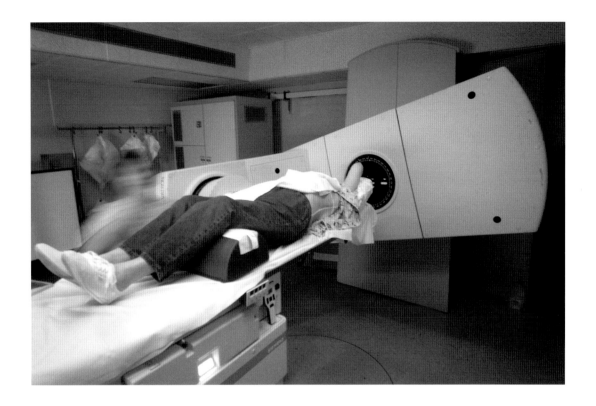

computerized axial tomography (CAT) and positron emission tomography (PET) scans and their respective before-and-after images simultaneously. Using one tool of the computer system, Dr. Rogers can literally trace the outline of the patient's tumor on the screen and measure its size to see if it has increased or decreased in diameter. Another function of the software allows Dr. Rogers to view the tumor in motion to see its growth or remission over the course of the patient's treatments. The tumor appears on the screen as a throbbing gray mass. It looks similar to a video game villain, but this evil creature is real—it lives inside Geraldine Thomas' body.

In his office, after meeting with Geraldine and viewing other patients' scans, Dr. Rogers uses various charts and formulas to calculate chemotherapy doses for patients. Each round of the cocktail of drugs is specifically tailored for each patient based upon weight and height. If a patient's body weight alters by 10 percent during the treatments, the doses need to be altered for the new weight. Any errors in calculations could have horrible results for the patients.

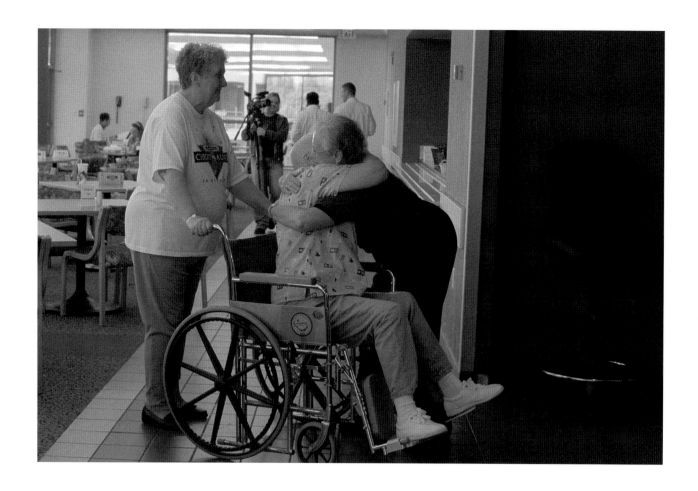

En route to the Rosenbaum Family House, Geraldine and her sister Mary stop to greet a friend who works in the hospital cafeteria. The House is a place next door to Ruby Memorial Hospital where adult patients and their families can stay for a small fee while loved ones undergo treatments. Because of her outgoing nature, Geraldine makes many friends among the patients, doctors and staff at the hospital during her six-week stay for daily radiation treatments.

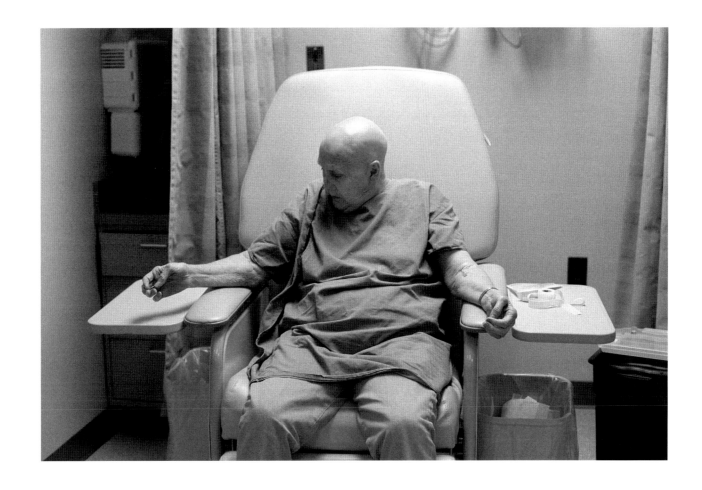

Awaiting a CAT scan to determine if treatment has shrunken the tumor, Geraldine wonders aloud which arm would be best for the intravenous port the nurses will install in her vein before the procedure. After examining the numerous scars from previous IVs, she gives up trying to decide. "They haven't told me anything about my chances yet," Geraldine comments, "but I reckon after all these tests is run, he will tell me."

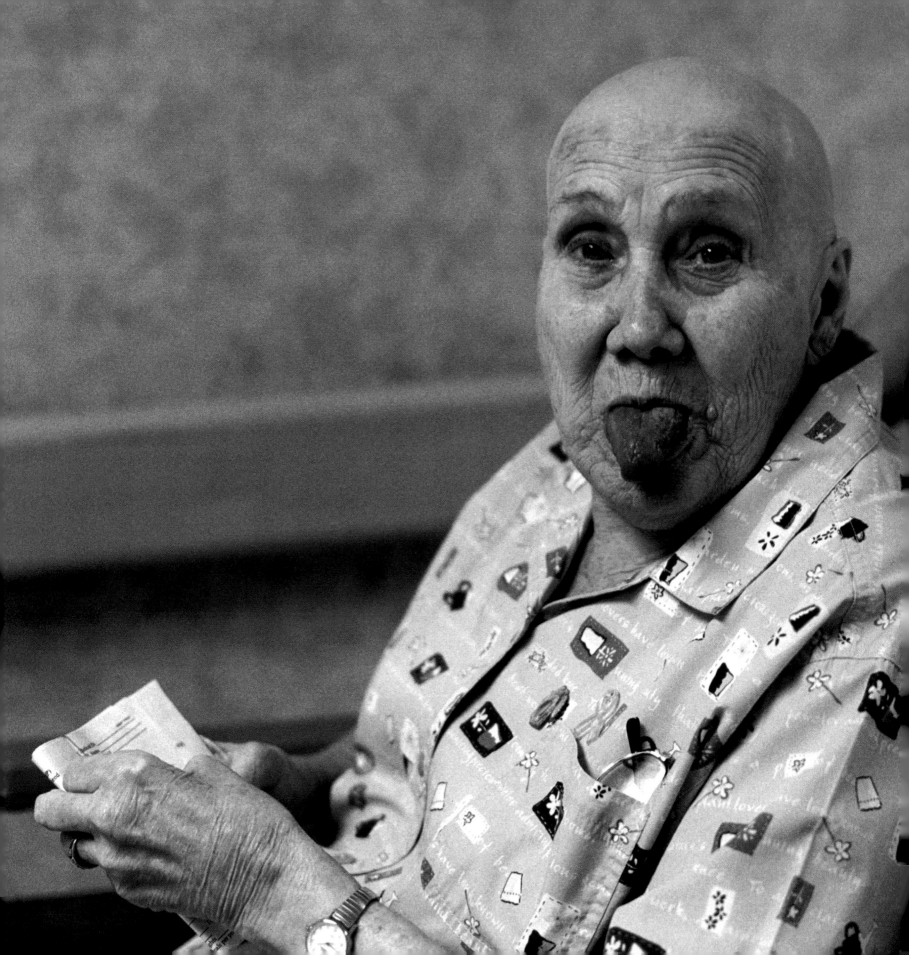

"We can go into a room, and everyone there will have a sour look. By the time we get to leave that room, everbody's laughing. We believe in laughter. It's good for you."

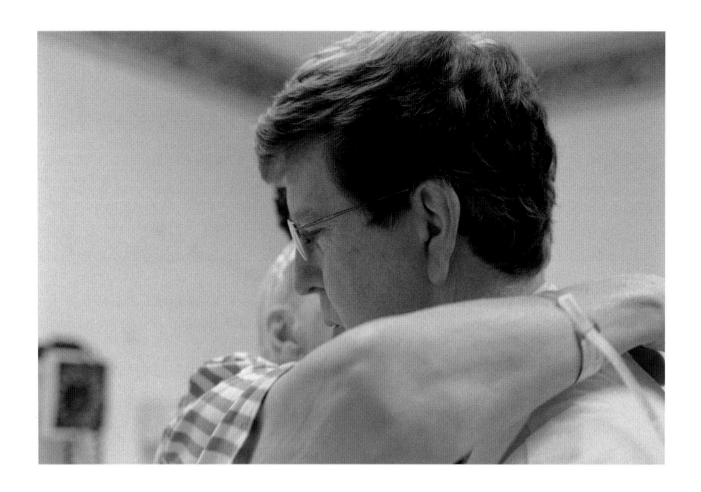

At the beginning and end of each appointment, Geraldine gives her oncologist, Dr. John Rogers, a big hug. This day, Dr. Rogers has bad news: despite chemotherapy and radiation treatments, the tumor has grown. He presents the option of discontinuing chemotherapy treatments, but Geraldine is determined to persevere and fight the disease.

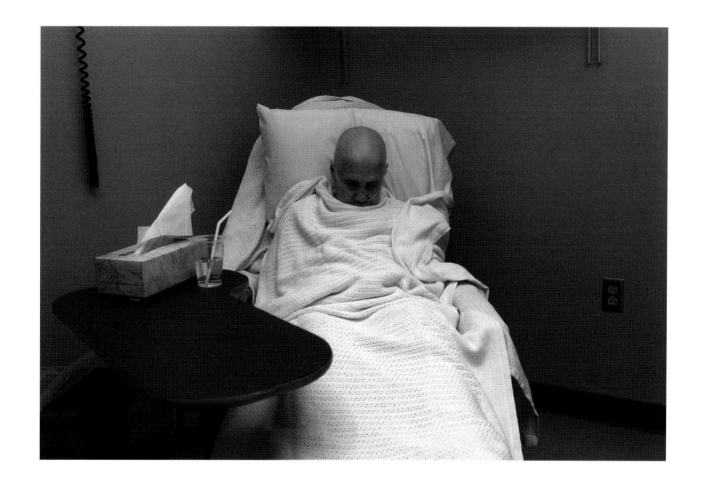

During a visit to the hospital in January, 2003, an exhausted Geraldine naps before a PET scan that will reveal pneumonia in both lungs and evidence of the cancer spreading. Because of the pneumonia, doctors were forced to discontinue chemotherapy. After this visit, Geraldine went home for hospice care and never returned.

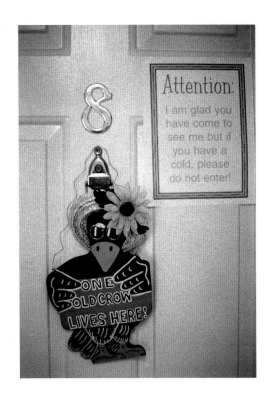

SEPTEMBER 2002

For her chemotherapy session, Geraldine walks to the rear of the center to an area that resembles an emergency room. Hospital curtains separate patients. She enjoys playing miniature video games, such as "Gone Fishin'," or watching television to take her mind off the treatments.

Geraldine wears two special pins on her flowered blouse to each chemotherapy treatment—both personal gifts from Brown. Resting on her lapel are a white ribbon, symbolizing lung cancer, and a golden angel with wings unfurled.

During Geraldine's first set of treatments, Brown wore the ribbon on her lab coat. When Geraldine asked about its symbolism, Brown removed the pin from her shirt and gave it to Geraldine as a special token.

"She wears that pin every day she comes to the Cancer Center," Brown said. "Even if she's wearing the most glamorous outfit, she still wears it on her lapel. Although it means a lot to her, it means even more to me, because I feel better just knowing that she's wearing it."

At her church in Summersville, Geraldine started a drive for supplies and clothing for the Cancer Center. After bringing numerous gifts from Summersville for Brown, Geraldine joked that Brown should return the favor by bringing her a box of chocolates. Brown vowed to remember the gift for Geraldine's next appointment. She wrote reminders on a half-dozen fluorescent-yellow Post-It notes and placed the sticky papers throughout her home so that she would not forget this important gift. As a result of Brown's persistent memory, the nurse practitioner presented Geraldine with another personal memento—a selection of Lindt truffles.

"She couldn't believe that I remembered," Brown said. "I don't think that she understands that she is always on my mind."

Geraldine's expressions are reminiscent of the slapstick comedians of silent films or vaudeville—she is always making humorous gestures to those roaming the halls. Her favorite? Sticking her tongue out at anyone who will watch. Geraldine's laughter, along with her banana bread, is her trademark, according to the medical staff.

"It's really common for us to ask of our patients, 'How are you feeling?'" Brown said. "But I'm slow sometimes when it comes to jokes, and Geraldine would always respond to this question, 'With my fingertips, that's how I'm feeling!' "

The 75-year-old makes continuous conversation and smiles to fill uneasy gaps of silence during her chemotherapy treatment. Today's topic: a reality show called "The Bachelor" that she had watched with her sister Wendy in the Family House.

She adds, "Who does that guy think he is? Having all those women and kissing them on national television?"

Geraldine is one of the most recognizable faces in the center. During treatments throughout summer 2002, Geraldine often wandered through Ruby Memorial Hospital's endless corridors, introducing herself to everybody.

After building friendships with the hospital's employees, on her first trip back to the center in autumn 2002, Geraldine was on a mission. Heading straight for the x-ray technician's help

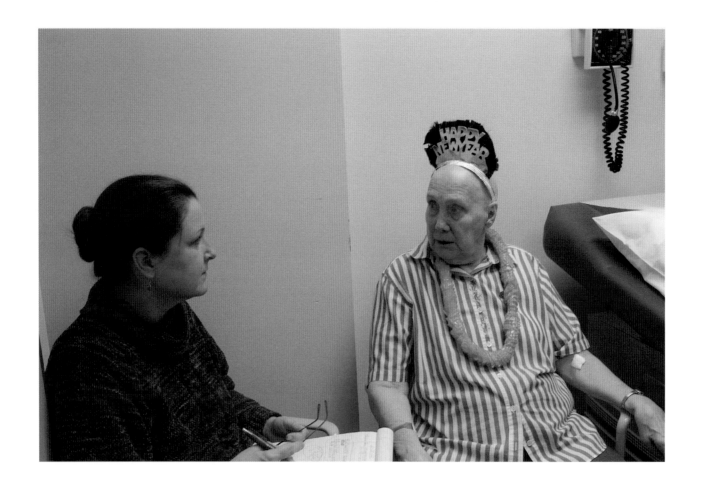

Shortly after New Year's Day, 2003, doctors are forced to discontinue Geraldine's treatments and arrange for hospice care at her home in Summersville. Despite several rounds of chemotherapy, there has been no success in shrinking the tumor, and her pneumonia has spread to both lungs. A social worker discusses hospice care with Geraldine.

desk, she stood politely behind the counter, waiting for the nurse to finish her telephone conversation.

She addressed her brief query to a nurse.

"That girl that worked here this spring, she's short and has, like, curly hair, did she have her baby?" Geraldine asked.

"Yes, ma'am. Beginning of July. She had a girl."

"All right," the bald-headed Geraldine stated with a laugh, as she clapped her hands in spontaneous celebration. "Cause I always went past here every morning when I stayed at the Family House and hollered at 'er. I remembered that she was gonna have a baby, and I just wanted to make sure that things turned out right."

December 2002

By noon, Dr. Rogers has examined 13 patients, prepared for his afternoon appointments, and studied follow-up labwork. Dr. Rogers' midday break is a working lunch. Sitting at his desk with a tape recorder, he dictates the morning's events for his notes. If he follows his schedule precisely, Dr. Rogers wraps up his duties at the Cancer Center around 6 p.m.

In the oncology profession, Dr. Rogers admits that it's hard not to take your work home with you—not only in your briefcase, but in your heart.

Dr. Rogers' confidence at the end of a day of facing grave topics, including mortality, stems from his steadfast faith in God, a force that guides his practice of medicine.

"It's hard to know that some of your best friends are going to die," Dr. Rogers said. "But before being a doctor, I'm a Christian first. It's important to place God first in this line of work. I want to let each patient know that they are special and that their time here on Earth is important. You don't want to have someone's life end and think that you didn't get to know someone."

His commitment to his faith is evidenced by the small poster that hangs from his private office door on the fourth floor of the West Virginia University Health Sciences Center. On the laminated paper reads the anonymous spiritual poem titled "Footsteps in the Sand."

Geraldine's son, Dana, is thankful for the influence of Dr. Rogers' faith in his practice and

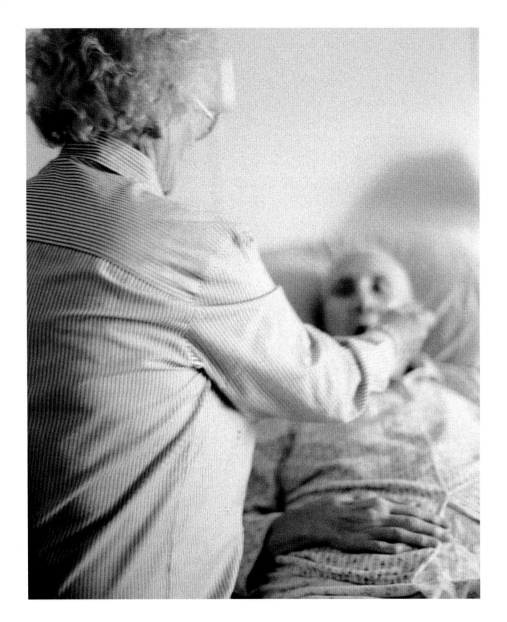

By early March 2003, Geraldine is at home confined to bed. A church member gives her spoonfuls of popsicle. To supplement hospice care provided by nurses, six friends from church take turns tending to her needs during the day, while her family members come over on nights and weekends.

on his team. "Dr. Rogers and the people he has, it wasn't like he was afraid to mention God. And I think that they rely on God, and that's been a real comfort to not only my Mom but to the rest of the family as well."

Although Vidya Brown does not share Dr. Rogers' Christian ideals, she relates that her work is a spiritual challenge.

"After working here, it's truly hard to believe in anything," Brown said, pressing her palms together in frustration. "But something keeps us going. I try to learn from my patients and keep hope alive. You can easily lose faith in this field because there are terrible events that occur without any real explanation that makes any sense."

Brown also asserts that it's difficult not to bring work home.

"Some days, you are just emotionally, mentally and physically drained by the time you come home," Brown said. "But I get energy and inspiration from people like Geraldine."

Brown agrees with Dr. Rogers' approach and displays her personal dedication by giving each patient her home phone number after the initial consultation. Brown advises those like Geraldine to call whenever they are in pain, feeling depressed or just need a warm heart to listen to their struggles.

"Geraldine calls me at home often," Brown said. "I feel like we have become friends through this. But I want her to know that she can call me and cry. She doesn't have to be upbeat and positive on the phone. Nonetheless, we have developed an extremely close bond."

Vidya Brown's helpline is not just for her patients; it's open for their families as well.

"Geraldine's son Dana has telephoned numerous times asking what he can do to ease his mother's pain. I'm there for any one of my patients like that 24 hours a day."

Reaching out beyond the traditional physician's swiveling stool, Dr. Rogers enjoys meeting patients' families.

"When you're talking about serious things—issues of life and death—you want to know that each person has a comfort-support zone," Dr. Rogers said. "Like with Geraldine, I feel like I've built a close relationship with her son, Dana. I know that she will be well taken care of."

"Geraldine just takes one day at a time," Brown said. "She has an amazing support system, and she's so courageous to try just about anything. We don't know if this new line of treatment will work, but she fortunately tolerates treatments very well. She knows her limits."

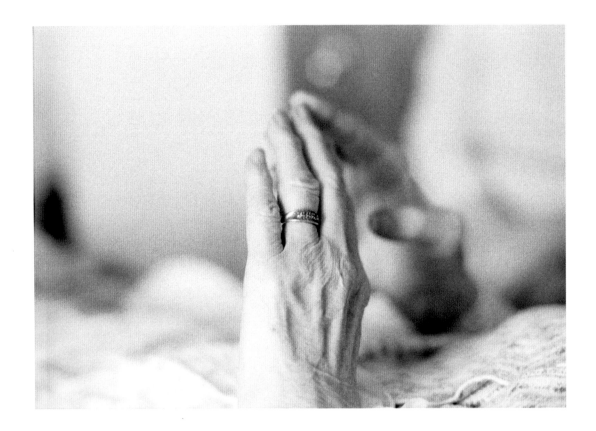

Dr. Rogers believes that her tumor has a 20 percent chance of decreasing but cannot promise that this round of treatments will cure Geraldine completely of the cancer.

"In Geraldine's case, no one really knows what will be," Dr. Rogers said. "As for now, she is not symptomatic from her disease, and half of patients respond well to this type of treatment.

"Patients typically go through diverse feelings in their treatment; ones of denial, anger, and then final acceptance," Dr. Rogers relates. "I think that's where Geraldine is now. She's found her peace."

Geraldine Thomas died in March 2003.

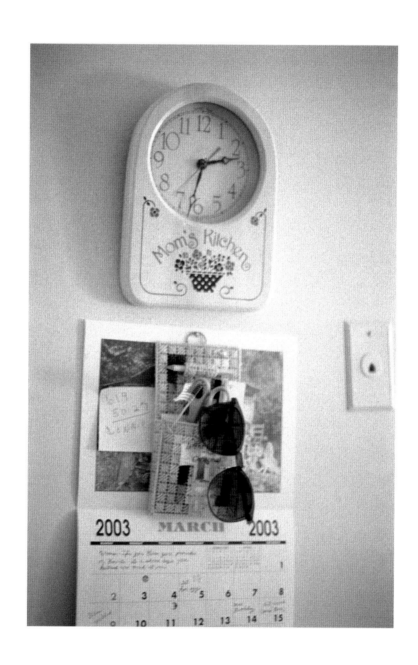

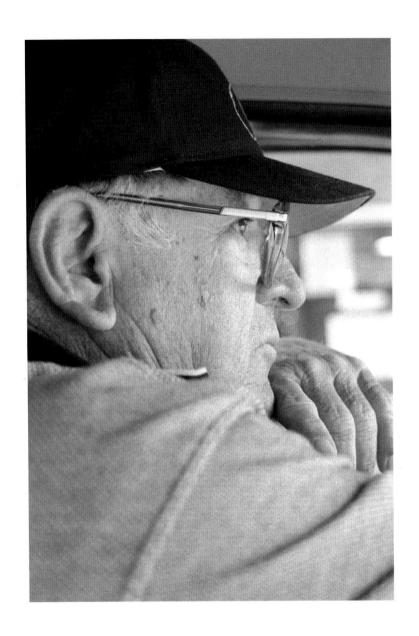

THE JUNCTION

text by KATIE STOUT

SEPTEMBER 2002

Things are quiet on this particular Saturday, as they often are in Shenandoah Junction. The clock at the Boyd household is just striking 2 p.m. Jesse Boyd sits in the rocking chair in the family room, and his wife Peggy is across the room beside the fireplace.

Behind Jesse on a cabinet are family photos and an old William Tell bank, along with pieces of antique glassware, two brass candlesticks, and several wooden cutouts of Amish buildings that Peggy purchased in Lancaster, Pennsylvania. She and Jesse have been to Amish country several times, Jesse says.

The mantel holds a plant and a metal replica of the statue of liberty that a neighbor brought back from New York for Peggy. Beside the blue plaid couch, there is a bookcase holding more family photographs and numerous books, including a book about purple martin birds and a book titled *The Great Tomato Patch Cookbook*. At this moment, Jesse and Peggy are talking about his diagnosis.

Jesse Boyd was diagnosed with acute myelogenous leukemia on December 6, 2001. Doctors caught his leukemia early and by chance while treating him for high blood pressure. After nearly 18 months, Jesse's cancer is still in remission.

photographs by KATIE STOUT

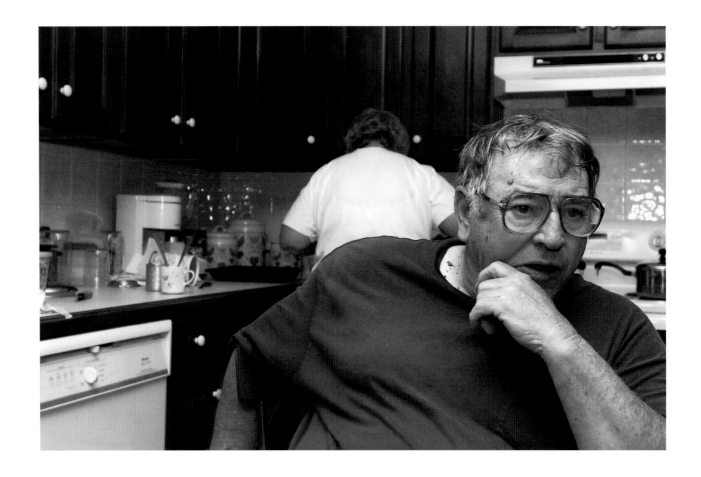

Jesse and Peggy Boyd first met in elementary school and have been married for more than 50 years. Their relationship is very close. "I would have taken it a whole lot harder if it had been her," Jesse observes.

"To be honest with you," Jesse says, "I just can't explain it. It just hit me so suddenly. I'm a deeply religious person, and I put it in the Lord's hands."

Jesse says that he was willing to accept whatever the Lord sent him. He often prays to get well. He also prays for others. The Lord's Prayer is his favorite.

"I would have taken it a whole lot worse if it had been her," Jesse says.

"Why do you say that, Jimmy?" Peggy asks, calling him by his nickname.

"Because. I would have," is Jesse's reply.

Nothing more needed to be said.

Jesse was diagnosed with acute myelogenous leukemia on December 6, 2001. He was 70 years old. His doctors caught his leukemia in its earliest stages, by coincidence, while treating him for high blood pressure. After doctors adjusted Jesse's blood pressure medication, he began to feel tired. He was weak and couldn't walk very far. He thought this was because of the new medicine. However, doctors began monitoring his blood every three months, and by the end of the year, they had detected leukemia.

The thing that surprised Jesse the most was the way he reacted to the news.

"I don't know why it was, but something was just telling me that it was going to be all right," Jesse recalls. "That's the only thing I can tell you. I just had as much confidence in the world that it was going to be all right. It never scared me. Now, I just tell you, it's amazing! I wasn't scared. It didn't bother me."

His life changed, of course, in outward ways. The trips to the Cancer Center. The treatments. But the basics remained the same. His marriage of 52 years. His sleepy hometown. His garden.

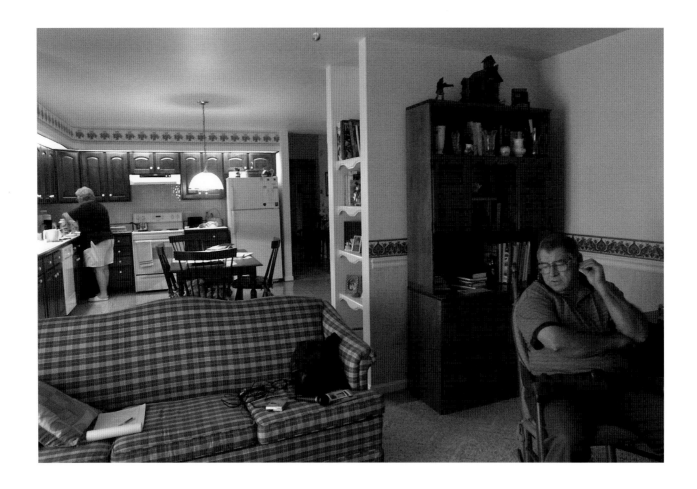

The Boyds are inseparable. While Peggy fixes a dinner of homemade beef stew, cornbread and fresh asparagus picked from their vegetable garden, the couple discusses current events. Every evening after dinner, they do the dishes together. Peggy washes and Jesse dries. "He says he doesn't know what he'd do without me," she observes.

Jesse's blood counts are still not back to normal. He is getting stronger, but his doctors had told him that it would take a year or more. Six weeks earlier, Jesse couldn't walk to the end of his yard and back without almost collapsing. Now, he is able to get around.

Jesse has color in his cheeks, and he has gained back the 35 pounds that he lost during his stay in Ruby Memorial Hospital in Morgantown, West Virginia.

"I wish I could have kept it off, but, she's too good a cook! And she likes stuff that I shouldn't eat. And that she shouldn't either!" They were both laughing.

Peggy and Jesse rise and go outside. They live in a ranch-style house on 2.44 acres, in a sub-development just outside of Shenandoah Junction, West Virginia. Out from their back porch is their purple martin birdhouse. They had four families in there this past summer. Jesse really enjoys watching them.

—·—

Peggy and Jesse met in elementary school. They started dating when Peggy was a junior in high school. They were married in a small ceremony two years later on March 11, 1950, in a parsonage in Hagerstown, Maryland. Peggy was 18, and Jesse was 19.

When Jesse was diagnosed with leukemia, Peggy was scared to death. It knocked her for a loop. Peggy says Jesse relies on her and that she keeps him going as well.

"He always says he doesn't know what he'd do without me," Peggy said with sadness in her voice.

However, Peggy says that Jesse is doing much better. "It was just the treatment that was so awful. That was the really hard part," she says.

"But, he's eating like a pig now!" Peggy says, laughing. "Both of us are!"

MARCH 2002

Jesse sits up in his hospital bed with one bare foot tucked underneath him. The chemotherapy has made all his hair fall out, and he is very pale. This accentuates the size of his ears and makes very obvious a few large moles above his right temple. He wears a white undershirt and plaid flannel pajama pants.

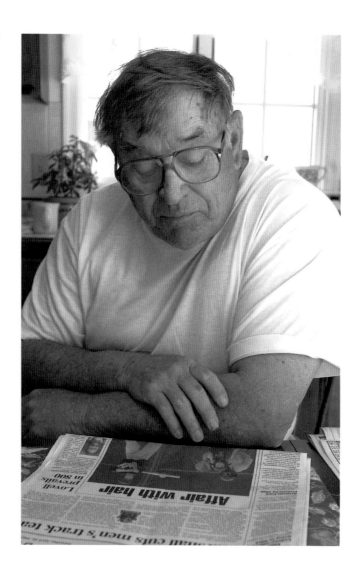

Most mornings, Jesse reads the newspaper to keep up on local events in Shenandoah Junction. Jesse dislikes the commercial development of West Virginia's eastern panhandle and hates to see corporations and chain stores pouring into the area he has called home for most of his 70-plus years.

When he sits up, he takes off his glasses. Now, maybe it's because he can't see very well without them, or maybe it's the chemo, but Jesse looks scared, vulnerable. He looks like a child against the stark hospital sheets, a look that is completely unlike him.

His voice sounds frightened as well, and sometimes he falters and looks toward Peggy to finish what he was saying.

However, the longer Jesse talks, the more comfortable he seems. Maybe talking about familiar things makes him feel like he's back home at the Junction, rather than in this hospital room. He begins to speak of the 42 years and four months he spent working for the Norfolk and Western Railroad, which is now called the Norfolk and Southern. He then moves to sports. He loves baseball. In fact, he played the outfield in high school.

"The [baseball] coach down at the high school sent me word over the weekend that he's holdin' me two season tickets," he says.

On the day that Jesse was born, his grandfather said that since Jimmy Fox had hit three home runs that day, he was going to call him Jimmy. So, since he was born, Jesse's family and friends have called him Jimmy.

Jesse was undergoing his third, and final, round of chemotherapy at Ruby Memorial Hospital. He had first come to Ruby Memorial in December 2001 and had stayed for 26 days. During seven of those days he received two different types of chemotherapy.

"Then you just have to set and wait for your blood cells to come down," he says. "Then, you have to wait for them to go back. After they thought it was safe for me to go home, they let me go for two weeks. Then I came back for a second series of treatments. Now this is the third."

Jesse's leukemia progressed rapidly, preventing his white blood cells from growing properly and fighting infection. These irregularly formed white blood cells were the ones Jesse's doctor first detected.

After that first round of chemotherapy Jesse went into remission.

"It's wonderful," he says. "Wonderful."

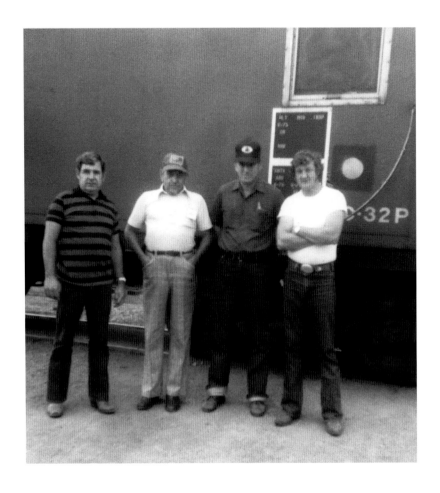

Jesse worked for Norfolk and Western railroad for 42 years and four months, mostly as a brakeman. In 1978, his crew posed for a group portrait at the yard in Hagerstown, Maryland. Jesse retired from the railroad in 1991. His father worked his whole life for the B&O railroad and died at age 84 from the same type of cancer that Jesse suffered. "In the summertime, those diesel engines, all those fumes blow right back into the cab of the engine," Jesse remembers. "You know it's not good for you, but what are you going to do?"

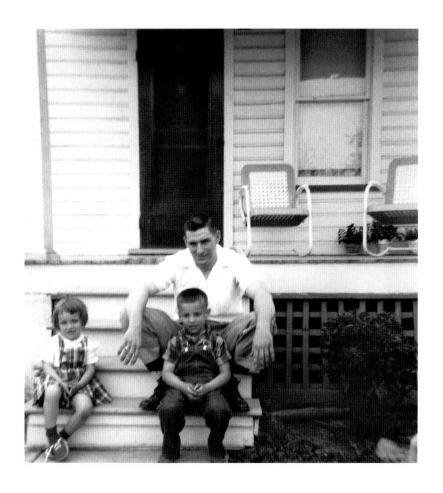

Jesse, around 1955, with his two oldest children, Carol Anne and Larry, on the porch of the house they lived in for more than 35 years. They eventually raised two more sons in the same home. Today, all four children and grandchildren live within 10 miles of their parents. There are few families in Shenandoah Junction the Boyds don't know.

Between hospital visits, Jesse returned to Shenandoah Junction, where he was born and raised. Peggy is also from the Junction. All four of their children and nine grandchildren live within a 10-mile radius.

The Junction is a sleepy little town in West Virginia's eastern panhandle, near Martinsburg and Charles Town. It is two hours outside Washington, D.C. You cross the railroad tracks and go around a bend in the road, and there sits the town's focal point, an old two-story house that is Shenandoah Junction's post office. Jesse goes there every morning, and it is there that he sees his friends and regularly swaps stories. The upstairs of the post office houses Shenandoah Junction's Masonic Lodge. Jesse is a member. There is also a grocery store and Jesse's church, the Shenandoah Junction United Methodist Church. However, Jesse says that a long time ago, back when the railroad was the main source of transportation, the Junction was a happening place. It is there in the Junction that the Norfolk and Western Railroad and the B&O Railroad meet.

AUGUST 2002

Jesse's blood counts are up to low normal. A normal white blood cell count can range from 4,000 to 10,000. At this time, Jesse's is closer to 4,000.

He still feels tired and draggy after taking his medicine. He mowed his grass today. His garden, which turned out four or five bushels of tomatoes this year, needs rain. His son, David, has already put up 30 quarts of spaghetti sauce from all the tomatoes. So far, he and Peggy have canned 14 quarts of green beans, and his lima beans are just starting to come in.

Jesse and Peggy climb into their white 1990 Cadillac Seville and go for a Saturday drive.

Going into the Junction requires them to pass the point where the Norfolk and Southern and B&O railroads meet. There, a family is stopped with their two children. Jesse says that people come from all over to watch the trains go by.

As Jesse and Peggy enter the Junction, they pass the spot where the old train station where Jesse started work used to stand. It is gone now. Weeds fill the foundation.

"Right there is where we went to school through the sixth grade," Jesse says, pointing out an old brick building. "It's not a school anymore. It's owned by the Ruritan Club."

Their church plans to make 85 to 90 gallons of apple butter to sell at a fundraiser. Jesse and Peggy have been busy washing quart jars, nearly 200 so far.

Driving through Charles Town, they pass the Edge Hill Cemetery where their parents and other family members are buried. That's where Jesse and Peggy will be buried. They already own plots.

Jesse didn't do anything different for his 71st birthday, March 16, 2002. He says he's still living the same routine.

On this day, he is sitting in the waiting room of the Mary Babb Randolph Cancer Center in Ruby Memorial Hospital talking to Peggy and his son, David. He finished his last round of chemotherapy back in January and is now only returning to Morgantown for routine visits. He is still in remission.

Some color has come back into his face, and all his gray hair has grown back. He is in good spirits. He's getting strong, he says. He's not as wobbly as he was a month ago.

He's changed his outlook on life, he says.

"I don't worry about things like I used to. I take each day as it comes," he says.

"I have a couple of friends that I was raised with, my age, that are worse off than I am with cancer. I feel fortunate. I feel like I'm lucky so far," Jesse says.

On this day, Jesse is grateful that he is doing as well as his doctors say. He is ready to accept his fate, putting it in God's hands.

"I've lived 71 years," he says. "If something should happen, I'm ready to go. I've got things in order. I don't want to go. I've got her (Peggy) taken care of. If anything happens to me, she doesn't have anything to worry about."

Jesse says he enjoys life more now than he did before he was stricken with cancer.

"I appreciate it more," he says. "You even appreciate the birds. We got a purple martin birdhouse in our back yard, and a couple new families moved in. And we watch them. Oh, they dart! You see them dart! They eat their weight in insects."

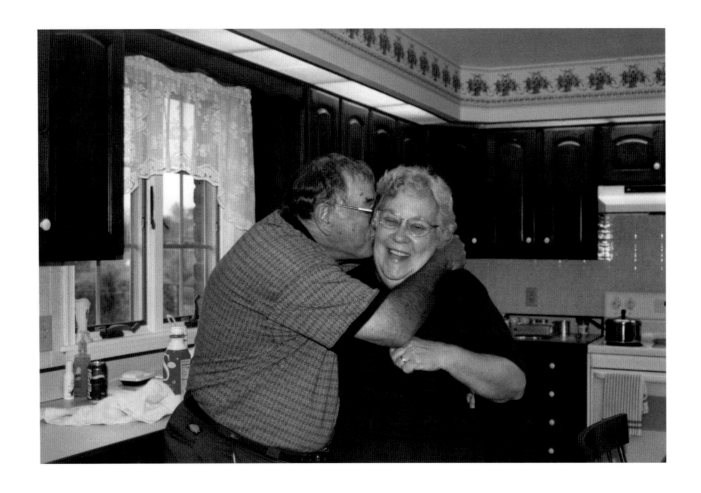

Jesse gives Peggy a kiss in the kitchen of their home. The couple first got to know each other in elementary school, married shortly after graduation from high school and have been together ever since. Besides their four children, they have nine grandchildren and three great-grandchildren.

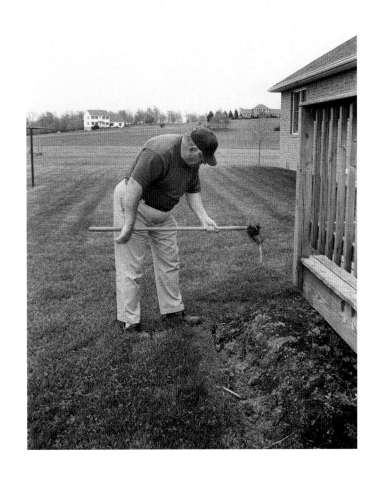

Jesse works in one of his flower gardens. In addition to roses,
he has a vegetable garden where he cultivates lima beans,
green beans, corn, tomatoes, turnips, kale, strawberries,
asparagus and raspberries. "I like to watch things grow."

"I like to watch things grow. Although, the frost killed my garden. Killed everything! I had to go buy new plants the day before yesterday. I have to start over again."

———

Arriving back home from their drive, Jesse settled back into the rocking chair while Peggy bustles about the kitchen making dinner—homemade broccoli soup.

He tells many stories of his friends from years past. He tells how he and Peggy's friend, Archie, had put mismatched siding on his house. He has himself laughing so hard a few times that he is nearly in tears. Peggy can be heard laughing from the kitchen.

APRIL 2003

Jesse and Peggy are still at home in the Junction. They still go sightseeing and to auctions. Jesse still piddles with his garden and runs his errands.

Currently, he is working on tilling the soil for his vegetable garden. He plans on planting a large garden again this year. His raspberries are already planted, and he's covered the small shoots with grass clippings to keep in the moisture.

Just the other day, Peggy made homemade beef stew and cornbread, and she and Jesse had guests over for dinner. They enjoy entertaining friends and family from time to time. Their youngest son, Mike, and his wife are living with them temporarily while their house is being built in Martinsburg.

Altogether, Jesse's lifestyle has not changed. There is still no trace of leukemia in his bloodstream. However, he still has to go back to Ruby Memorial Hospital every six months for routine check-ups. Jesse is past the highest risk time period. He has been in remission for one year and two months.

As for what his future holds, Jesse has "put it in the Lord's hands."

"I don't worry one bit," he says. "I take things one day at a time."

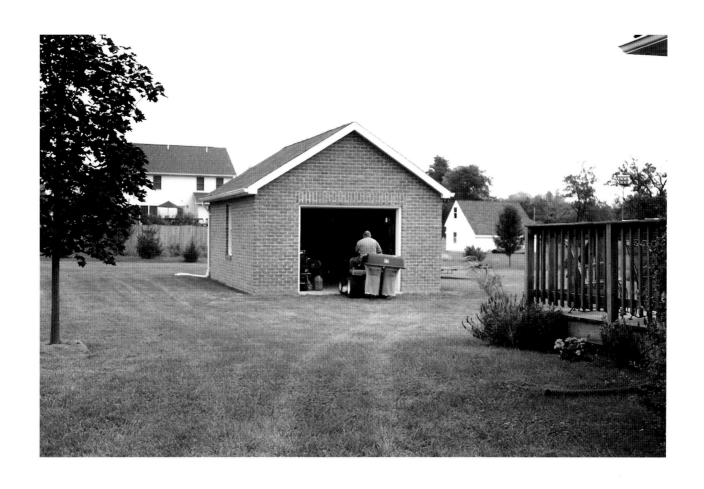

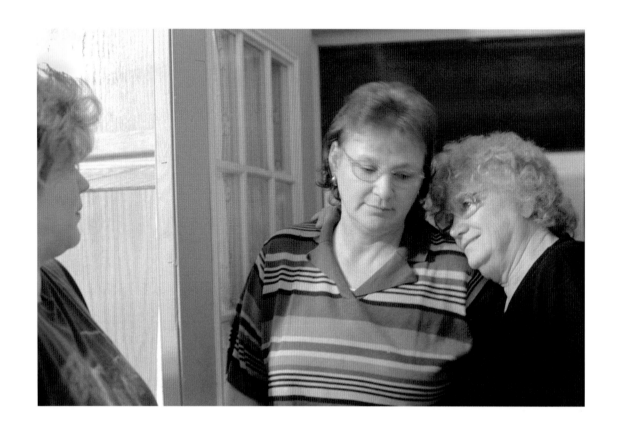

REMISSION

text by KELLY CARR

Brenda White pulled herself into the passenger seat of her red Jeep Cherokee. Her red shirt and pants matched the color of the vehicle and her gold earrings signified the importance of the day. The ride was different this time—so much so that there wasn't anything to say. The noise from the wipers removing the drizzling rain was the primary sound. As the Mary Babb Randolph Cancer Center appeared in her view, Brenda began to take deep breaths. Since being diagnosed with ovarian cancer more than seven months ago, she had been waiting for this day.

"Well, this is the last one," she said as she struggled out of the Jeep and shut the door. Walking toward the hospital, Brenda felt a mixture of anticipation and fear. She continued to take long breaths, hoping to calm her nerves. She looked at the rows of empty chairs in the waiting room and finally chose one. In an attempt to change her focus, she took out a copy of *Chicken Soup for the Mother's Soul*. She knew the waiting-room routine. Her husband took his usual place in the chair next to hers. Two other companions accompanied them, hidden deep in Brenda's pocket.

"Brenda White," the nurse called into the waiting room. The voice had the patient

In November 2003, Brenda White was living on the other side of cancer. Having completed all of her treatments, she was in her 15th month of remission from ovarian cancer. Remission, however, did not mean that Brenda's life was back to normal. She now faced medications to treat nerve damage and the fear that the cancer would return. Above, sister-in-law Sherry and Sherry's mother Marie tell Brenda how important it is to take her recovery one step at a time.

photographs by BARBARA GRIFFIN *and* MELISSA NETHKEN

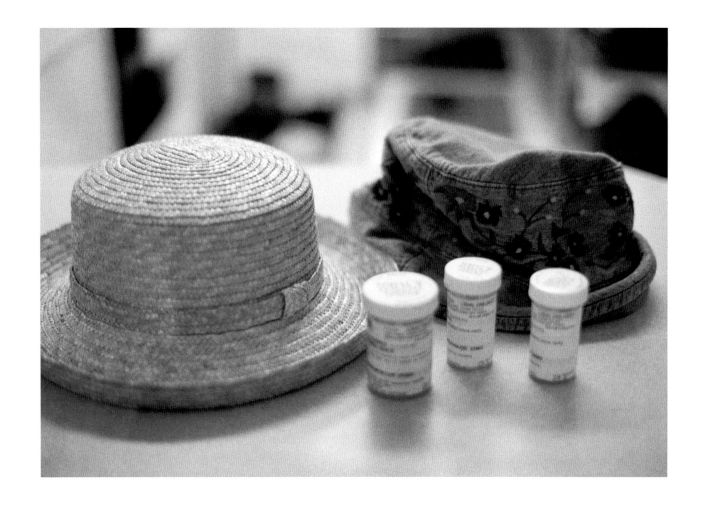

Even in remission, Brenda has constant reminders of her ovarian cancer. Brenda wore many hats when she was undergoing chemotherapy. "Hats are OK, but you can still tell you are bald," she observes. "Every time you go to the restroom it is a constant reminder that you have cancer."

instantly on her feet. The nurse pulled on green gloves and began undressing Brenda. She started at the collar of her shirt and rolled it down. Half of her chest, which included a port, was clearly visible. It was the channel through which chemicals flowed into her bloodstream. You could see it under her skin; it was shaped like a stethoscope. She never thought she would have a piece of metal implanted in her body. But this fact and being exposed in front of strangers didn't seem to bother her. From numerous doctor appointments in the last year, she knew if being exposed was the worst part, it was a good visit. "This is my last one. This is my last chemo," she said to the nurse for the third time since entering the room.

———

Almost eight hours later, chemotherapy already seemed a distant memory. She was confident as she approached the exit doors. For her, it was the last walk, the last mile. Balloons, flowers, and a bottle of champagne awaited her in the parking lot. Joe had the bottle in his hands, while his wife waited with a plastic cup. He struggled with the cork—celebrations of this kind are rare for the Whites. Brenda and her husband wrapped arms to taste the champagne in unison.

"This is nasty," Brenda said after her sip. "It must be an acquired taste."

Patients continued to file in and out of the Cancer Center doors. The Whites were alone in their party.

Brenda reached into her pocket and pulled out her other support system. To each chemo session she had carried two silver angels for hope and strength somewhere in her pocket. When she was first diagnosed, words like hope and strength were something she questioned. Now, her confidence in them beamed through her bloodshot eyes. "I carried these with me to every treatment," she said. "Now I am going to put them away. If I ever need them, I'll get them out again."

On this day, the angels seemed to have done their job. But soon she would seek them out again.

———

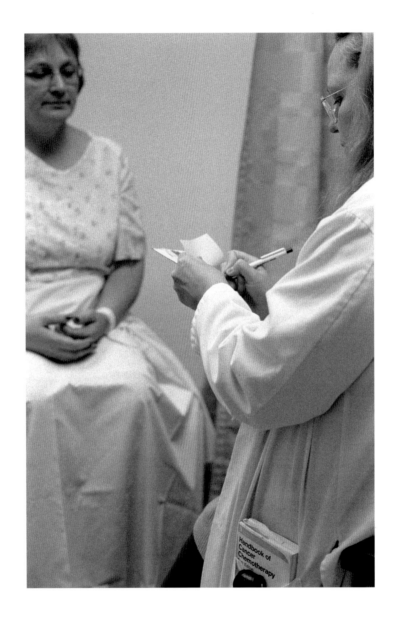

Routine medical exams are needed to continue to stay cancer-free. November 2003 marked Brenda's second year since being diagnosed with ovarian cancer, and her 15th month in remission.

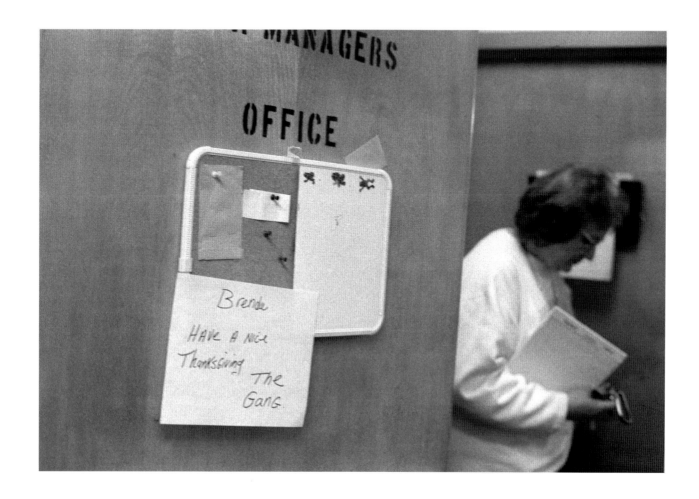

Brenda, who is a building supervisor on the downtown campus at West Virginia University, works during Thanksgiving because her staff is off for the holiday and the first week of hunting season. The long hours leave her exhausted, but Brenda never gives up, keeping her job throughout the trying months of treatment and recovery.

At first, Brenda had thought it was a pulled stomach muscle. During routine house cleaning, the vacuum, as usual, was being difficult. No matter which way she maneuvered it, the sweeper couldn't reach into spots Brenda wanted to clean. Unable to fit it behind the bed, she called her husband, and they moved the bed into a better position. The house was spotless the next day while Brenda sat at the doctor's office. She was diagnosed with a persistent ovarian cyst, which led to a hysterectomy. After the surgery, she was scheduled to go to the fifth floor, but she never made it. Alone in her hospital room, she felt frightened but relieved.

"At least it's not cancer," she thought.

Everyone in the family knew the truth but her.

———

Now—at the visit for her last chemotherapy—she was cancer-free. Her oncologist, Andrew Soisson, MD, at the Mary Babb Randolph Cancer Center, had given her a pelvic exam and a blood test. Both revealed no sign of cancer. Those words are what registered in Brenda's head. She believed those words signified an end. But the exact meaning of "cancer-free" can be confusing for patients. Some choose to ignore the facts while some just don't understand.

"Cancer-free" is what the tests tell Dr. Soisson, but he knows cancer can return. He wasn't lying to Brenda when he said she didn't have cancer. But he often finds himself dangling between offering facts and encouraging hope. "You can't lie, but you don't want to rob your patients of all hope," he explains. "You have to explain the situation as accurately as you can. They have to know what the term 'cancer-free' means and that the tests have inaccuracies. You tell them the truth, what is on the exams and x-rays. They can be cancer-free at that point, but how likely is that the truth?"

———

"Remission" is a term that refers to the response of a cancer to treatment. It does not mean that the disease is cured. In order to deem a patient "cured" or "cancer-free," time is a crucial factor. In most cases, a period of several years without a recurrence is considered a good sign. Ovarian cancer patients often experience a relapse in the first two years following treatment, but the cancer may also return years later. Early ovarian cancer recurrences usually generate no symptoms. Follow-up care is a key defense to ensure survival. Around her fifth treatment, Brenda believed herself closer to the end than she actually was. She was braver and more curious than before. She read statistics as if they no longer applied to her. The average life span of an ovarian cancer patient was the topic that caught her attention. "Five years," she said to herself. "How could that be possible?" Reality set in—five years wasn't long enough. She wanted to live. She wanted more time to be a grandmother, a mother, and a wife. Brenda ended her quest for knowledge as quickly as she began it.

Brenda thought her problems with cancer would end altogether with her check-up. After that visit with her oncologist, she felt confident and energized. She was ready to reclaim everything cancer had stolen from her: seeing basketball games, watching her grandchildren, walking outside. A list had already begun to spin in her head. But Brenda didn't anticipate how hard the escape would be. How long it would take to feel healthy. How long it would take to stop feeling like a cancer patient.

She knew she had just one chemotherapy treatment to go. Then it would all be over. Her doctor said she was cancer-free, that her tests had said it for a while. She knew she had to finish one more chemo, but it was just a precaution. She assured herself that she had a clean bill of health. Brenda relayed her good news to other cancer patients. She felt badly that they would still be sick, but she still felt excited for herself. The conversations, however, offered more than she anticipated. Some patients were back in for treatments because of a second or third relapse. A few were clearly losing their battles. It became obvious that she was only in remission, that she wasn't as "cancer-free" as she believed.

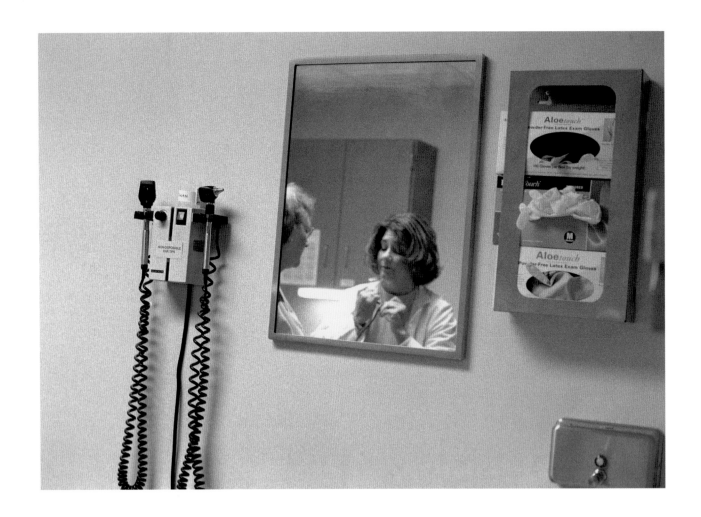

Routine medical checkups not only help Brenda stay physically healthy, but they also give her peace of mind. "The term 'cancer-free' is very deceiving," she muses. "It seems like a false sense of free health."

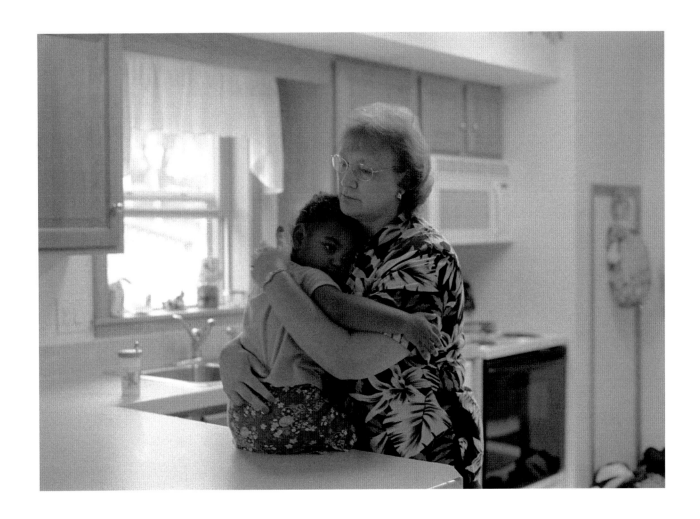

After battling cancer, Brenda's life has changed dramatically. Brenda, who once obsessed over a clean home and keeping everything in order, now puts her family first. On a day off, she takes time to hold granddaughter Dominique.

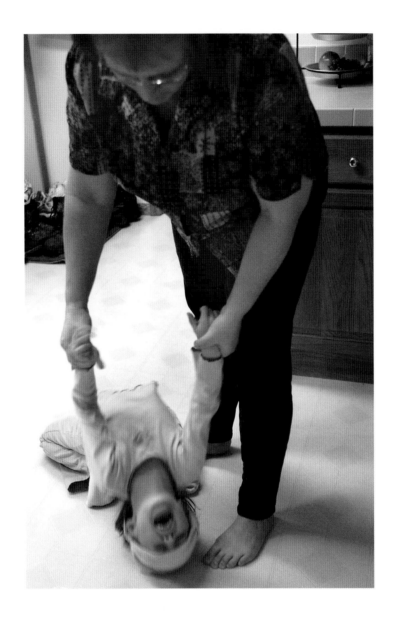

While the cancer is in remission, Brenda has the strength to play with her grandchildren. During a family cookie-baking session where the children each wear one of her chemotherapy hats, she has fun with granddaughter Bailey.

When she was diagnosed, living without cancer seemed so far away. But now, after her final chemotherapy, it seemed a reality. Her first goal was to return to work. With her husband on disability from his job as a coal miner, she had taken on the responsibility of earning their sole income. Cancer had put her work in West Virginia University Housing on the back burner. Fighting the disease was difficult; managing finances was sometimes more challenging. She had tried working four hours a day throughout her illness, but her body lacked the strength it used to have. The chemicals from chemotherapy lingered in her system, sending shooting pains through her arms and legs.

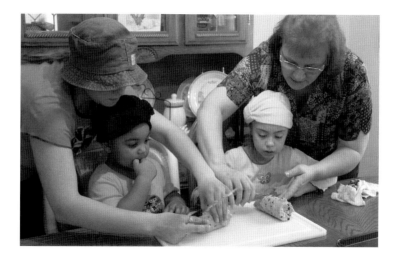

After her first round of chemotherapy, she developed a hatred for mirrors. Even in her house, she would try to ignore them. "It wasn't as bad looking at myself with a wig on, but I tried not to look without them," she says. "As long as I didn't see it, I didn't feel any different." Instead of losing strands of hair as she anticipated, she lost clumps. At times it was almost impossible to drain the tub. The hair wrapped itself around the soap and lingered everywhere on her body. It took three days for her hair to fall out completely. Her first round of chemotherapy had ended, but the side effects had just begun. Bloodshot eyes, yellowed skin, and hair patches were now part of her attire. "For three days I tortured myself," she said. "Watching it fall out day-by-day is too emotional. I would advise anyone to shave it, cry, get over it, and move on."

———

"Hats are OK, but you can still tell you are bald. I think the hair issue is the biggest one for women. Every time you go to the restroom it is a constant reminder that you have cancer. Your body doesn't feel that way at all except during the treatments."

It could be just a look or a tone of voice. No matter what it was, it was different. The way people addressed her, the way her family talked to her—nothing about it was normal. She was not just Brenda. Now she was Brenda with cancer. She wasn't watching the kids or mowing the lawn. She wasn't grocery shopping or cleaning. She wasn't the one to call anymore if you needed a favor. Cancer changed all that. Everyday there were "those" phone calls. People wanted to know her progress, but unlike before, their voices were softer. The conversations were never confrontational or complaining. Instead, most were a formality with the same script. There were things her sisters stopped telling her. Conversations were held behind her back about her condition. Problems were dumped onto other family members. They were selective with what they would tell her. She craved an argument. She wanted to yell. If just one person would battle her, she wouldn't feel like a cancer patient. She wouldn't feel like she might die. But every visit and conversation was as fragile as possible. Her body was drained from the acting, the pretense from both herself and her family. "I knew things that would trigger them. I knew if I lay down too much they would worry," she said. "I tried to say up longer and longer so they thought I was getting better."

Recovering from the chemo was taking longer and longer. After her third treatment, she became accustomed to the limited diet and lack of comfort. As Brenda tossed and turned on the couch searching for a position, Joe would bring her a Popsicle. "Your whole body aches like a toothache," she says. "It would be nice if you could sleep, but you can't really sleep."

She'd flip through the channels hoping to find the Montel Williams Show. It's her favorite show, but she could only focus on it for a few minutes at a time. The pain under her arms and in her legs would break her attention span. On post-chemo days she didn't change out of her pajamas. She took pain medication, ate crackers and drank Ensure. The nausea and vomiting made her feel flu-sick. She found herself listening to the background noise of her family rather than to the TV. You could tell when it'd been four days because she'd have traveled to the living room. For the first three she did not stray far from her room. Going to the bathroom was her only activity, and she liked being alone. "This stops your life and makes you do some soul searching," she says. "You begin to realize what is important. The best thing to do on these days is to lie in one place, and then sit for a while. You change positions a lot."

It was after the fifth treatment that she wasn't sure she could do it anymore. By the third day she knew she would be in bed longer this time. The pain had spread everywhere, and the nausea was unbearable. It was summer, and her family was enjoying the weather. Last year, she was outside playing with her grandchildren. This year she had to settle for hearing their laughter from her room. "Oh my goodness. Is it going to be like this until the end?" she thought. After each chemo she would mark the calendar with her recovery days. This time, the duration had surpassed that of any other treatment. Usually it took four days; this time she realized it would be seven or eight. She tried to remember if she'd ever felt sick from cancer. To her it always seemed as though it was the cure that was making her sick. Her friends' calls were what kept her going. They told her she was going to make it, and she chose to believe them.

Her set date to return to work was August 19, just three months after "cancer-free" entered her vocabulary. That day she returned for the full eight hours. A short time into her day, she realized things were quite different than before. She couldn't be on the floor, working with her staff. She couldn't climb stairs or lift objects. As the woman in charge, she found herself losing control. Cancer was still affecting her, and remission was turning into yet another battle. "I believed it would get easier," she said, "but then I started to ask, 'when?' When could I walk farther than across the kitchen floor? I set such high expectations for myself, and I couldn't meet them. I was so excited about getting better that it kind of overwhelmed my common sense." The fight to survive was over, but reclaiming her life had just begun.

She found herself once again pulling out the angels. She picked them back off her dresser and placed them in her pocket. "I remember walking over and putting them in my pocket," she said. "After the second day of work I started falling apart. I needed all the strength I could get." She thought the angels had done their job, but she soon realized that yet another battle had begun.

Her doctor said the effects from chemotherapy would last 30 days, but it had been several months since her final treatment, and the effects were still lingering. She had talked to herself throughout her illness, but now the conversations were more frequent. "I would tell myself, 'I am going to do this'," she said. "As I got stronger, I would make a goal to do something every day by myself. I couldn't run the vacuum, but if I saw something on the floor I would get it with the Dust Buster. I would think 'I got a crumb. I did something to help.' Everyone wants to nurture you, but you have to get off the couch and fight." At work, she started giving herself more orders than her coworkers. "It's OK. It's all right," she told herself. "It's only the side effects of the chemo. I'm not getting worse. Baby steps, baby steps."

The internal chatter became a constant habit that kept her sanity together. On this particular day of her first week of work, Brenda had to open the door to several dorm rooms. The staff was asked to place refrigerators in each. There was no manual labor involved in her task besides carrying the key, which itself didn't appear heavy. She walked up the stairs to the first room and opened the door without a problem. The next one was a little more difficult—she was slower on the stairs and behind the rest of her staff. On the second flight she felt herself almost collapse. By the third room, her exhausted body gave up. She wondered if everyone was like this.

After her second week of work, she couldn't get out of bed. Brenda was responsible for two buildings, and each required a quarter mile to walk. Before cancer, she would walk the buildings three times a day. Now, she couldn't even imagine doing it once. She wanted a date when she would be normal again. When she went to work, it compromised the rest of her day. She immediately came home at night and collapsed. The next morning, once again, she was forcing herself to shower. Getting dressed and the drive alone exhausted her. Still, she refused disability and catastrophic leave. Work was supposed to get her life back on track. It was supposed to be one thing she could control. Instead, working became a constant reminder that she was still a cancer patient. One hour in her workday felt like eight. The escape she expected wasn't that at all. She thought working would signify the end of her struggle, but it did just the opposite.

Losing her hair was one of the most difficult side effects. She quickly added hats, scarves and wigs into her wardrobe. "You look like a man, but you're still my grandma," Brenda's granddaughter said. At work, her bare head deeply concerned her. She began to notice her staff was troubled as well. No matter how healthy Brenda looked or how productive she was, her head was a constant reminder of her struggle. She had shared the experience with her staff since her diagnosis. They made visits to the hospital and called her at home. It was Brenda's lack of hair, though, that seemed to make cancer a reality. Without something to cover the chemo's damage, it made some uncomfortable. "One of the ladies' moms died of breast cancer, and I think it just brought back too many memories for her," she said. "I had a lot of hot sweats, and I would have to take my hat off. When I did it, I just made sure I was in an area where no one could see me."

A girls' day out with members of Brenda's family helped to ease the shock of her hair loss. It was a Saturday, and her sisters went on an adventure to Chic Wigs. After paying a five-dollar deposit, everyone scattered through the store to pick out a wig. Brenda's mother and mother-in-law assumed the position as judges on a bench in the hallway. "We would walk out, and they would say 'no' or 'yes,' whatever they thought," she said. "We spent the entire day doing that."

Curing Brenda's appearance insecurities snowballed into more weekly events. Her family decided spending time together was a top priority after her diagnosis. There were no two weeks alike throughout her illness. The sisters had beauty parties and produced a show for her brother's 40th birthday party. They ate cake for Valentine's Day and went out for danishes. "Before I was sick I would say 'I'll do the dishes, and then I will call my sister,'" she said.

"Now I check on my sisters, and the dishes wait. I think life moves so quickly we just get our priorities mixed up. Things happen, and you realize washing down the walls isn't as important as going on a picnic."

Brenda's ranch-style house, tucked at the end of a gravel driveway, has a modern but comfortable appearance. Her grandchildren's toys scatter the sides of the living room. A flowered couch, where she sometimes rests, is placed in perfect view of the television. There were some days, when searching for understanding, she would read about cancer. But as many times as she did, Brenda would never read past the pages describing her stage of cancer. For her, the unknown was better left that way. She had tried a few times, through other patient's stories, to understand her future. In the end, it only created horrid premonitions. "I got to this one part in a book I was reading and thought 'Oh, my God'," she said. "I walked straight over to the trash can and threw it away. I just had to get rid of it. I had to put it some place where I didn't have to think about it."

The book was called *Nancy's Journey: A Feisty Cancer Story*. Nancy Lofstead, a West Virginia woman who battled ovarian cancer, was the author. It was a gift from her sister after her diagnosis. At first, she believed it would give her insight on what she was up against. Brenda soon realized that she had to set page limitations. "I got the book and read three or four chapters, and then I had to put it down," she said. "When it got farther into the things she went through, I was not ready for it. When I got to that part myself, I would pick the book back up and take the next step." Months later as she sat in her living room, Brenda believed she could handle the conclusion. Over the last year she was careful, only reading books with positive outcomes. Now cancer-free, she felt she could manage anything. She gave old pamphlets and brochures a second glance. *Nancy's Journey* reappeared in her hands as well. This time when she picked up the book, though, things were different. She was reading the material with a new set of eyes. In her mind, cancer was over and she now read as a survivor.

Finally, she could read the end. As a "cancer-free" woman, conclusions were no longer scary. "I thought, 'OK, I am cancer-free. Mine was a happy ending, so I am ready to cope with this,'" she said. "At the end of the book she was not cured, and I was shocked.

"It was a reality check. The term 'cancer-free' is very deceiving. It seems like a false sense of free health. Using the word 'remission' is probably better. Now I know I'm really not cancer-free until it is gone for five years."

Brenda realized that there had to be something she could do differently at both her job and in her life. There had to be another way to make things work. There had to be a simple solution. She didn't want sympathy, just her life back. She knew she could call her staff if she needed them. The constant reliance, however, was exhausting to her. She was the one that had cancer. She felt guilty forcing everyone to accommodate her disease. She understood that she still had a long way to go, but she had never realized her life was this physically demanding. Neither her staff nor her family minded the change, but she still sometimes felt like a burden. The change, however, worked for her. Brenda had changed and so had her life. Everyone else had accepted it long before she did. Now both she and the people surrounding her have embraced the change.

Brenda was in her backyard, trying to help her husband and his friends build a deck. Although they didn't particularly need her help, she wanted to contribute anyway. Brenda confidently lowered herself underneath a piece of wood and threw her arms up. The small task made her feel included, like an active participant again. It was a day where she could have done a hundred things if she'd had the energy. She could grocery shop. She could cook. She could clean. Everything Brenda had been dying to accomplish suddenly filled her head. "For right now," she thought, "I'll just help with this." Just as quickly as Brenda volunteered, just as soon as she began feeling useful—it was gone. She couldn't breathe, and her sides hurt. Again she was in pain. Again she was back at the hospital.

The first thing that came to her mind was cancer. "Maybe it came back," she thought to herself. "What if I have to go through all of this again?" There was, however, a simple explanation for her pain. From all the chemicals injected in her system throughout her illness, her muscle tissues were soft and sensitive. She had pulled several of them. Brenda couldn't help but smile when she thought of herself holding her breath, believing the battle with cancer could start again.

But that's the way it is. Every little thing, every day scares her. She tries as hard as she can to not let the idea of cancer dominate her life. Sometimes, though, it is hard. Brenda has learned that it will always be a part of her life in some form. She has learned to accept it, instead of fighting against it.

EPILOGUE

After 18 months of remission, Brenda White's cancer returned.

She felt certain the cancer had come back even before her doctor confirmed that a tumor had emerged in her abdominal area. In November 2003, she felt lower back pain, then cramping and fatigue. She even noticed a strange body odor. A nurse later told her that she was very in tune with her body.

Because the tumor was not attached to a specific organ, surgery was not a good option. The doctors scheduled Brenda for six chemotherapy treatments.

Before one doctor's appointment, Brenda sat with her family and discussed how she was coping. She pointed to her head.

"The battle is up here," she said. Then she pointed to her stomach. "Not down here."

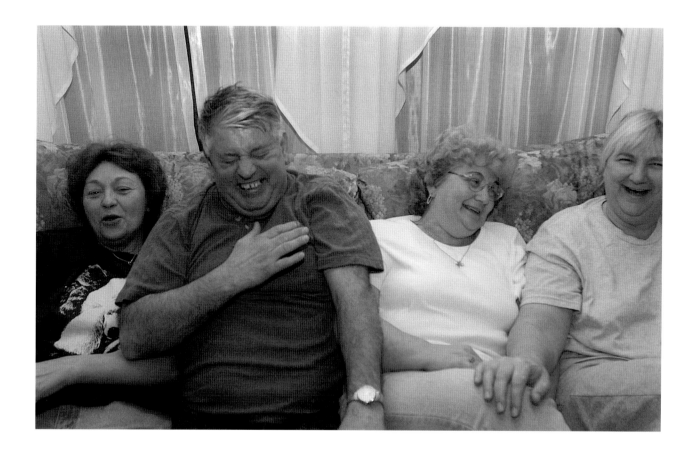

With the news that Brenda's cancer had returned, her family gathered around to give their support. Her sisters, Betty Golden, Barbara Golden, and baby sister Pat Mason, along with Brenda's husband Joe, not only provide Brenda strength, but they also share with her their own form of healing: laughter.

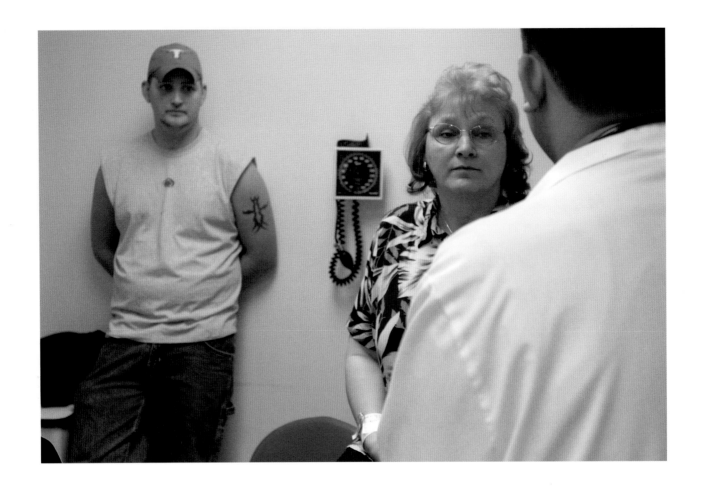

Brenda returns to the Mary Babb Randolph Cancer Center for an appointment with Dr. Eddie Reed. He discusses her treatment options and answers questions from Brenda and her family. Her son, Butch, came along to find out why her cancer was inoperable. After having his questions answered, he expresses confidence that his mother is in good hands.

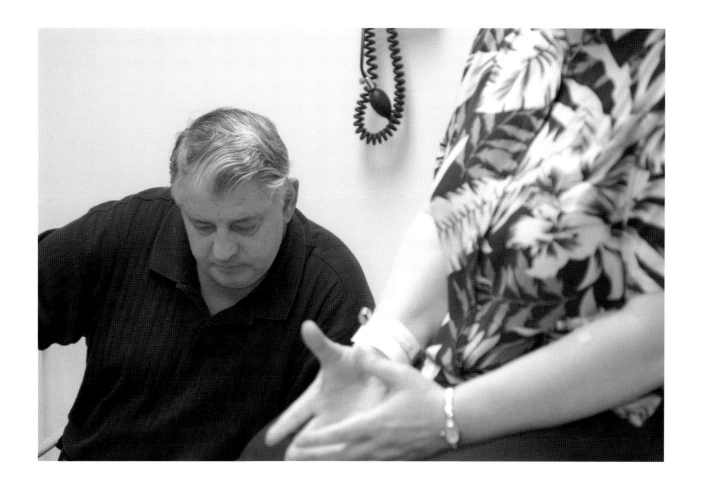

Brenda's husband Joe is the one who will take care of her as she begins to battle cancer once again. He listens quietly as Brenda describes to her sisters how she knew the cancer had returned months before doctors diagnosed it.

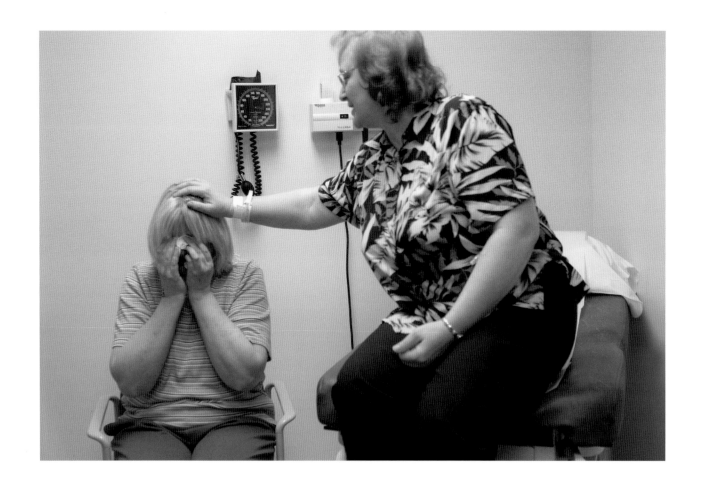

Along with her son and husband, Brenda's three sisters also came to her appointment. Having heard that the treatment Brenda would be receiving was not to remove the inoperable cancer but to control it as long as possible, her sister Pat breaks down and cries. Brenda remained calm and comforted her.

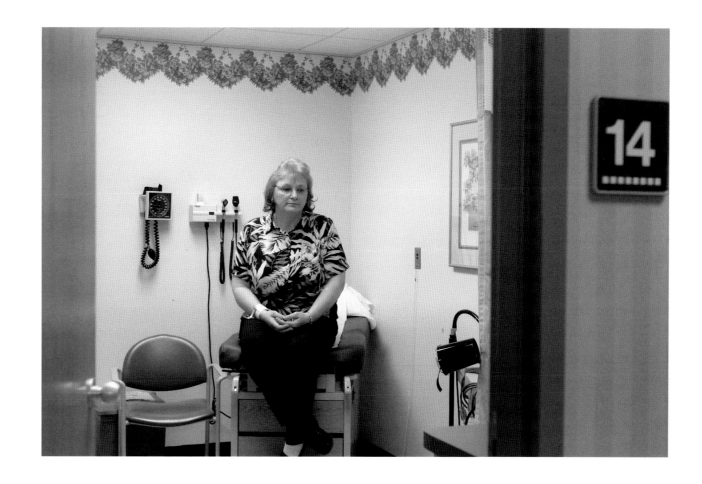

With the return of the cancer, Brenda's worst fears have been realized. She knows her biggest fight is not with the cancer but with herself. "The battle is up here," she says, pointing to her head, "not down here," and she points to her abdomen.

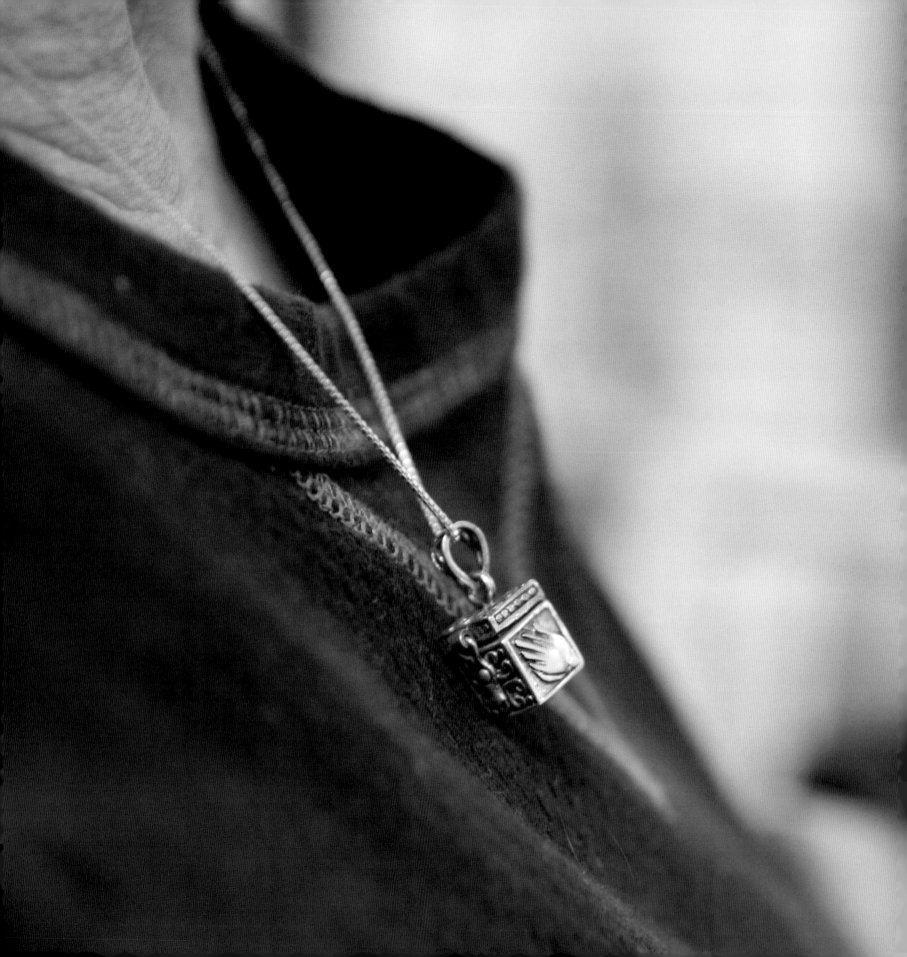

"If you have faith as a mustard seed,

you will say to this mountain,

'Move from here to there,'

and it will move;

and nothing will be impossible for you."

— MATTHEW 17:20

Brenda's sister Betty wears the prayer box necklace she bought for each of her four sisters upon hearing the news that Brenda's cancer had returned. She's placed a mustard seed in each box with a verse from Matthew 17:20.

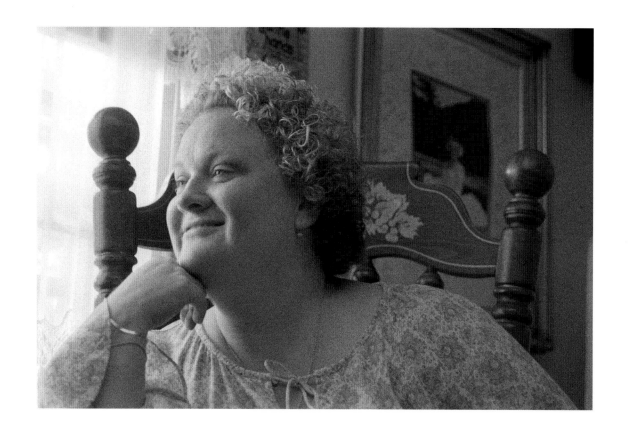

STUBBORN ENOUGH

text by PAM KASEY

Cindy Drummond lay on a wheeled cart, curly red hair in a ponytail, trying to warm herself under a thin, white blanket. The sealed sterility of the surgical holding room offered no hint of the rising November sun. Cindy fired instructions at her boss.

He needed to gather the x-rays for the surgeries he would perform the next day. He had to look through the patients' charts to review their physical exams, since she wouldn't be there to pull them out for him. Their histories, too. And he shouldn't forget to check if any had abnormal lab results.

Richard Douglas, MD, stood in green operating room scrubs holding Cindy's right foot in support, listening, a little amused. Finally, he had to ask.

"Did you or did you not have Versed?"—a pre-surgical sedative.

"Yes …"

"Well damn it, you need some more," he said. "You're still giving me orders!"

Dr. Douglas, a neurosurgeon, had recruited Cindy as his nurse two years earlier for just this quality: her ability to manage under pressure. She'd worked in intensive care and had a good

---

Cindy Drummond, 34, was diagnosed with breast cancer November 26, 2001. Cindy is a clinical nurse specialist at the West Virginia Neurosurgery and Spine Center in Clarksburg, West Virginia. Being in the medical profession gave Cindy a different perspective once she was diagnosed. "It's more difficult now for me to deal with patients with breast cancer, but it's made me a little more understanding."

photographs by COURTNEY BALESTIER

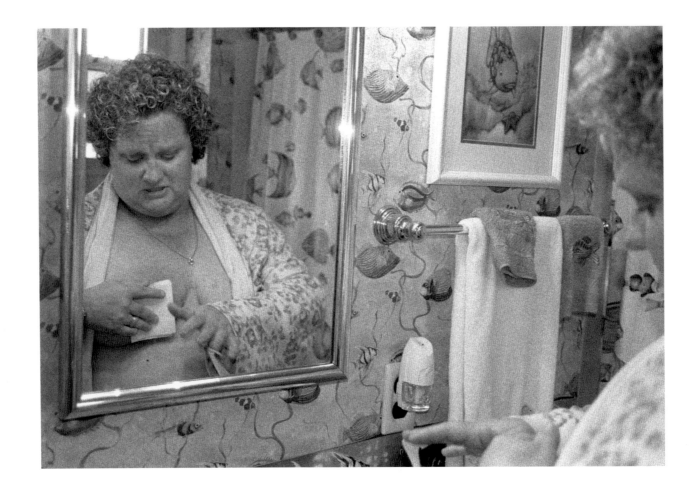

Infections have caused Cindy to redress her wounds several times per day, usually in full view of her children. A large plastic box sits beside the bathroom, holding her gauze, disinfectants and Clorox bleach. "They always hug me from the right side," she said. "They'll ask, 'Does your breast hurt?' You can't keep stuff from them. They know everything."

reputation. He respected her work and taught her as much as she wanted to learn. They'd become friends. Their families cheered together at West Virginia University football games. Dr. Douglas and Cindy's husband, Kevin, had taken up archery together and planned to go bow hunting.

And over the summer, Dr. Douglas and Cindy had competed to see who could lose 50 pounds first. He'd won, but she'd found a lump in her left breast, a lump she'd been unable to feel when she was heavier—a lump that should have been nothing at age 32. But the radiologist who'd read her mammogram the previous Wednesday rated it "category V, highly suspicious."

The radiologist, unable to get through on Cindy's line, had called Dr. Douglas, as she'd requested. Dr. Douglas had reacted quickly. As a neurosurgeon, he primarily saw patients with back pain, but the ones he saw with cancer had it bad: advanced cancers that had spread to the brain or spine. Even before talking with Cindy, he'd phoned Thomas Kennedy, MD, a surgeon whose office was two floors up, and gotten an appointment for her that same afternoon.

Dr. Kennedy had told her the lump was too big and varied for him to perform a biopsy by needle. It really had to come out. The sooner the better. First thing Monday.

Cindy had dreaded this surgery every minute since, though she'd pulled herself together to cook Thanksgiving dinner for 11 the next day, then suffered through the long holiday weekend. She'd spent hundreds of hours in the OR, but she had never gone under general anesthesia herself. She was scared. She'd asked Dr. Douglas to assist Dr. Kennedy, a request that surprised and gratified him.

Cindy had also asked Karen Abruzzino, the scrub nurse that she and Dr. Douglas usually worked with, to help. Karen came now with a scrub tech. They wheeled Cindy feet first through big double doors into Operating Room 12, the newest operating room at Clarksburg, West Virginia's United Hospital Center.

It was Cindy's first time here lying down. She looked around. An anesthesia cart stood ready, and tables nearby displayed sterile instruments on blue cloths. She scooted herself onto the black vinyl operating table in the center of the room. Cold, all but naked, she squinted under the round adjustable surgical light. She'd never realized how bright it was. Cindy expected there would be music later—she thought Dr. Kennedy probably liked classical—but the room was silent now.

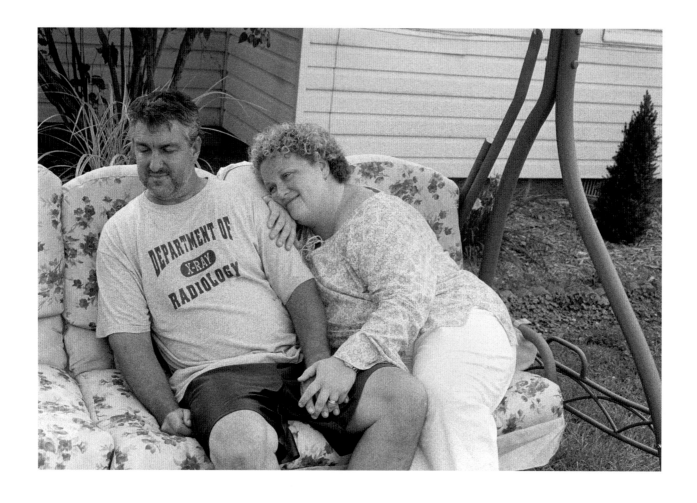

Cindy says she feels her bout with cancer has strengthened her marriage. "It's made us way closer," she says. "Kevin missed some karate. He didn't go on a baseball weekend with his friends. But he didn't miss one chemo treatment."

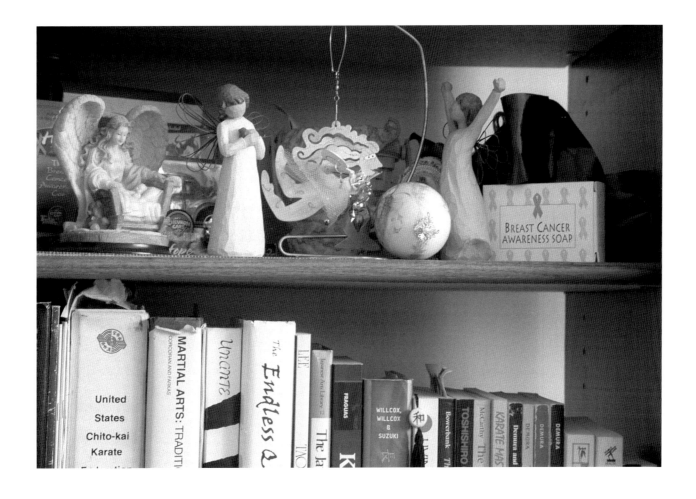

Through her months of cancer treatment, friends and family have given Cindy dozens of tokens, trinkets and ornaments. Below her collection of angel figurines, breast-cancer awareness soaps, and hand-painted goose eggs sits the small library of books Kevin accumulated on Eastern and alternative medicine and therapy. "I never really looked at them," she admits.

Dr. Douglas held Cindy's hand until she realized that Karen was about to prep her. "He has to leave now!" Cindy protested. "He's not going to see my boob!" As Dr. Douglas stepped out, Karen prepared to swab Cindy's left breast with brown-orange Betadyne disinfectant and drape her for surgery. A nurse anesthetist brought a clear rubber mask over her face, and Cindy thought of her boys, Elijah, just four, and two-year-old Noah … would she ever see them again?

After surgery, Cindy awoke in the recovery room. She felt better than she expected, considering Dr. Kennedy had carved a four-inch-diameter chunk from her left breast: the lump and a margin of healthy tissue all around. They wouldn't know if it was benign or malignant until the following day. Kevin took her home. She slept.

———

Cindy had succeeded in getting pretty much everything she'd wanted in life so far. She'd decided as a young girl to follow her older cousins into nursing and went straight from high school to nursing school at West Virginia University in Morgantown, an hour north.

Then she set her sights on Kevin. He was a mechanic at the local airport where she worked part-time to put herself through school. He had hair down to the middle of his back. He rode a motorcycle and studied karate. They became friends, going to WVU football games together. He loved the red curls she'd always hated, and convinced her to grow her hair long. They dated.

Cindy accepted an offer from WVU's hospitals when she graduated. She worked long hours in intensive care and felt most satisfied when she could help the sickest patients. "Just don't tell me I can't do something!" she liked to say.

When Cindy and Kevin married and started their family, she knew she'd have to cut back her hours at the hospital. Then Dr. Douglas approached her about working with him at the West Virginia Neurosurgery and Spine Center near their home in Clarksburg.

Dr. Douglas was a formal dresser whose charms included a tendency to switch between his professional and goofball personalities mid-sentence. Cindy liked him immediately, and his medical practice was perfect for her. A former Marine who'd married a third time in his mid-40s and had a daughter Elijah's age, Dr. Douglas held fairly regular office hours. He often worked evenings, but not too late. He challenged Cindy by teaching her and by encouraging her to take classes to become a nurse practitioner. They were different—he the pessimist, she the optimist; he the procrastinator, she the bustler—yet similar, and considered themselves alter egos of each other. Mrs. Douglas would come to call Cindy her husband's "work wife."

Cindy was dressing Tuesday morning when Dr. Douglas called.

"I have to go to Kennedy's office," she told him. Dr. Kennedy was going to give Kevin and her the biopsy results, but she suspected Dr. Douglas had already seen them.

"Yeah, I know."

"Yeah, I know you know. Are you going to tell me, or what?"

"Dr. Kennedy's your physician, he told her, and you need to discuss this with him.

"But you're my friend," she argued. "You tell me."

Finally he gave in. "It's not good. It's medullary carcinoma."

"What the hell does that mean?" she blurted.

Dr. Douglas wasn't familiar with the term either. But they both knew it meant cancer.

———

Dr. Kennedy invited Cindy and Kevin into his office, where he had met with her the week before. Oak shelves lining the room held titles like *Cleft Palate and Cleft Lip* and *Operative Hand Surgery*. A wall of windows overlooked the hospital. Dr. Kennedy, tall in spite of a slight stoop, kept his desk in order and gave his time and attention generously.

Cindy and Kevin listened as Dr. Kennedy explained that medullary carcinoma is rare, accounting for only five percent of breast cancers. It's usually slow-growing, the cancer to have if you're going to have breast cancer. He told them that Cindy would need three doctors for the three phases of her treatment. Dr. Kennedy would remove lymph nodes from her armpit in a second surgery. After that, she would see a medical oncologist for chemotherapy. And at the end, a radiation oncologist would give radiation treatments. The doctors would work together under the medical oncologist, so she should meet the others as soon as possible. Kevin wanted to know about the long-term, and Cindy asked Dr. Kennedy outright if this cancer was going to kill her.

It wouldn't, he told them—not if he had anything to say about it.

Kevin was fixing dinner, and Cindy had changed into her sweat suit and was taking a break from the phone that evening when Dr. Douglas called. He'd done some research since morning. It looked to him as though she had a long, debilitating treatment ahead of her. He was calling in part to say he understood that she was going to have to stop working.

"Stop working …?"

"Stop working."

Cindy couldn't believe what she heard. Her feelings were hurt: He'd underestimated her. He'd scared her, too. She'd worked continuously since she was 14 and loved this job more than any she'd ever had. She was nothing if not a nurse. She paced her kitchen floor as she heard Dr. Douglas wonder how anyone could take her place.

They argued.

She snapped, "When you're ready to deal with this, you let me know!"

She hung up.

The phone rang and rang. Friends brought food, flowers, balloons, chocolates.

Cindy needed sleep.

———

Wednesday morning was cold and dreary, but Cindy arose optimistic. Today, she would meet her medical oncologist, the person who would hold it all together. He would help her keep working.

Noah stayed with Kevin's mom and dad, but Elijah understood that his mother was sick and wanted to be with her. At the oncologist's office, they took seats in the waiting room.

Cindy played with Elijah. She read him all the kids' books in the magazine racks. Kevin walked Elijah up and down the hall, and a while later they walked together again. Other patients came and went. It was getting late for lunch.

Eventually, a nurse took them back to an examination room, and they settled into the two side chairs. Elijah sat patiently on Kevin's lap.

Finally, the doctor entered. He didn't offer a hand, or apologize for being late. He took a stool on the other side of the exam room. He flipped through Cindy's chart, then examined her breast quickly, giving a cursory description of the chemotherapy he expected she would receive.

Cindy asked for details about the treatment. He told her she didn't need to worry about it. She asked about side effects, and he told her she didn't need to worry about them either. Her most important question—Can I continue working?—got no real answer at all.

Leaving the office, Cindy felt like she would be dead the next day. The doctor had spent no more than 15 minutes with them. Just because she was a nurse didn't mean she understood everything about chemotherapy! How could she go through months of difficult treatment with an oncologist who refused to answer even basic questions?

Working in intensive care, Cindy had seen nurses and doctors make split-second decisions every day. She had a good idea what mattered in a medical professional. Credentials, sure. Skills, of course. But at least as much as those qualities, heart. She worked at that in herself all the time: Had she spent enough time with that patient? Had she listened well enough? Could she have been kinder?

Dr. Douglas was the same way. While in the Marines, he'd been hooked up to a ventilator for several months after a staph infection destroyed a large part of his lung capacity. His heart had stopped two separate times, and doctors had not expected him to survive. During his worst nights, one of the interns in the hospital sat by his bed and held his hand. Dr. Douglas finally began to recover. He felt inspired by that intern to study and apply to medical schools from his hospital bed, driven to pay society back for his life. When a general visited to invite him to stay on in the Marines, Dr. Douglas responded, "Sir, I have another mission in life."

Just as the intern had done for him, Dr. Douglas gave special attention to his patients. He liked to spend a little extra time and joke around with them, keeping each patient's hope alive in any way he could. Every once in a while, he would take a steak dinner to a patient who was bedridden.

Cindy didn't know who she would turn to now, but there was no way she could go through chemotherapy with this oncologist.

———

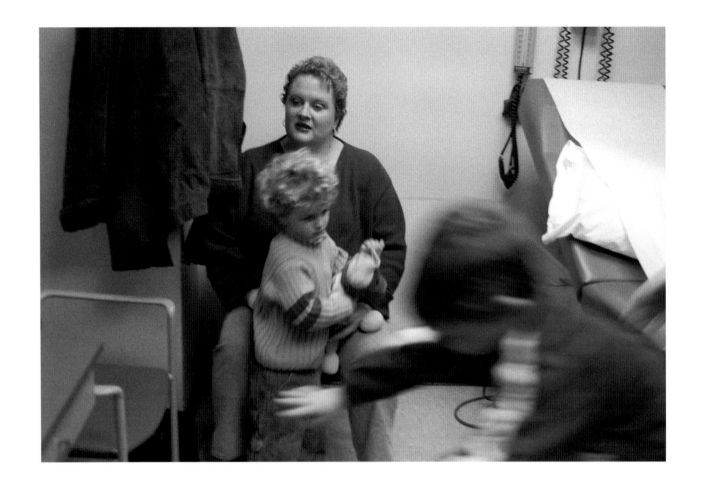

Cindy talks to Kevin while sons Elijah and Noah play in the examination room at the Mary Babb Randolph Cancer Center in Morgantown. She is waiting for her oncologist, Dr. Jame Abraham, to arrive for a routine exam. "None of them have sugarcoated anything," Cindy says of her doctors. "Dr. Abraham will tell you straight up."

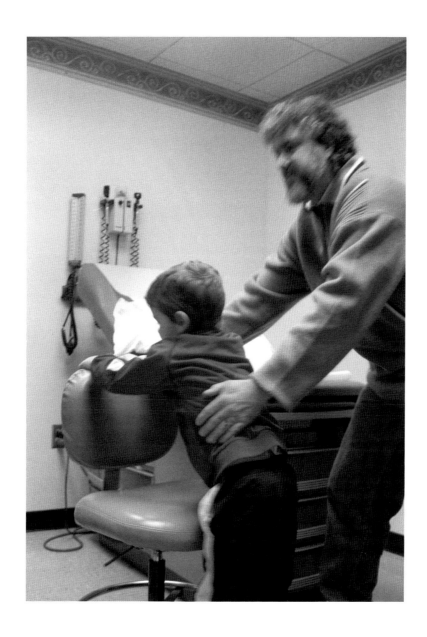

Kevin corrals son Elijah while the family waits to see Cindy's oncologist.

Cindy returned to work Thursday, worried about finding a medical oncologist and still furious with Dr. Douglas. The first patient she saw needed to have staples removed. As she began removing them he asked her, "What are you doing here? Dr. Douglas said you were never coming back!" That did it. She had to prove him wrong.

Being a cancer patient dominated her free time. Cindy decided to make an appointment with a medical oncologist at her old hospital in Morgantown. She met with a radiation oncologist, Scott Watkins, MD, an open, knowledgeable man who patiently answered her questions. She had a CT scan to check for the spread of cancer to her organs and a bone scan to check for spread to her bones. Both thankfully negative.

She and Kevin answered phone calls and gratefully accepted more meals from friends than they could eat. When she could, Cindy, still recovering from her surgery, slept.

———

The following Wednesday, Cindy and Kevin drove to Morgantown to meet with medical oncologist Jame Abraham, MD. Cindy hoped he would be the doctor who would work with Dr. Kennedy and Dr. Watkins to coordinate her treatment. She had dressed for the season: a red v-neck sweater and red socks decorated with snowflakes.

Dr. Abraham walked out to the Cancer Center waiting room to introduce himself to Cindy and Kevin before her appointment. "I'll Be Home for Christmas" played in the halls as he and his nurse arrived to meet them in the exam room a short while later. Slight and dark, soft spoken, with fine south Indian features and subtle expressions, Abraham quickly found a connection between himself and Cindy: He had a two-year-old son as well.

Abraham scooted his stool close to Cindy and asked her how it was that she'd come to see him. Her story gushed out: the lump she'd discovered in the shower, the mammogram and surgery, the doctors and scans. She explained about the medical oncologist she'd seen and how he'd told her she didn't have to worry about anything. "I don't need you to sugarcoat it," she said. "I just need to know that you're going to answer my questions."

He asked about her personal and family medical histories, looking for anything that might explain why a woman so young would get breast cancer, or anything that might indicate whether the cancer had spread. Dr. Abraham also wanted to understand her state of mind. As a medical student, he had helped an aunt live with, and die from, ovarian cancer. That experience and many since had taught him that mindset affects the course and outcome of treatment.

Then he asked his nurse for a sheet of yellow lined paper from her pad and began sketching and scribbling his way through five main considerations that drive treatment decisions. He wrote:

> SIZE — The size of the tumor, Abraham explained, gives a first approximation of seriousness. At three centimeters in diameter, Cindy's tumor was not small.
>
> LYMPH NODES —The number of lymph nodes involved helps to indicate spread. Cindy's lymphectomy was scheduled for January, so this was still unknown.
>
> ER / PR —Biopsy tissue with estrogen or progesterone receptors suggests that the cancer will respond to hormone therapy, improving the prognosis. Cindy's tumor was ER- and PR-negative.
>
> CELLS —Here Abraham drew a series of four pictures: a circle in a rectangle, a circle in a slightly warped rectangle, and two more versions. The last one looked like a fried egg. Cancer cells that resemble normal tissue look like the first picture. They are termed "well differentiated," and tend to grow slowly. Poorly differentiated cancers, like the fried egg, more often spread quickly. So much for having a slow-growing cancer: Cindy's cancer cells were poorly differentiated.
>
> HER-2/NEU —Over-expression of this gene causes a tumor to grow fast. Cindy's tumor showed normal levels.

Several factors worked against Cindy: the size of the tumor, the lack of hormone receptors, and the poor differentiation of the cells. Dr. Abraham recommended a standard chemotherapy regimen: four treatments of Adriamycin and Cytoxan—"AC"—spaced three weeks apart, with the possible addition of four treatments of Taxol, depending on the outcome of the lymphectomy.

Dr. Abraham discussed the side effects of chemotherapy, writing on a second sheet of paper.

Chemotherapy attacks cells that reproduce quickly, not only cancerous cells but also the stomach lining—leading to nausea and vomiting; the blood-producing cells in bone marrow—increasing risk of infection, tendency to bruise and to heal slowly, and fatigue; and, of course, hair follicles—causing hair loss.

In spite of the side effects, he told Cindy, patients do best when they maintain as much normalcy as possible in their lives. Cindy blinked back tears at that, dabbing delicately at the corners of her eyes with a forefinger. He gave her the yellow pages of notes. He and his nurse would be in touch with Dr. Kennedy and Dr. Watkins; they would see her again in January, after her lymphectomy, and she could call any time.

She and Kevin walked to the car. "I think everything's going to be okay, now," Cindy said as they drove home.

It had been two weeks since her mammogram, two weeks since she'd relaxed. She had her team of doctors. Now, well, there was everything else.

———

That's how it was, in the beginning. Cindy just did the things a cancer patient has to do: recover from surgery, get scanned, find doctors, keep people informed. She was tired, but she didn't think of herself as a sick person. After all, she was young, and she'd done everything a woman can. She'd had her kids in her twenties and nursed them both, in part for the protection against breast cancer. She didn't feel sick; she felt good. Having lost that weight the previous summer, she looked good, too.

Cindy found herself identifying with a breast cancer patient who came by the Spine Center in January, not long before she herself was to start chemotherapy. She and Dr. Douglas first met Rebekah in October. Rebekah was 43 years old and had been treated for breast cancer six years earlier. The cancer had returned in her brain and paralyzed the left side of her body. Dr. Douglas removed the tumor, and she regained nearly all of the use of her limbs. Now, in January, Rebekah looked vigorous, trim and tanned. Dr. Douglas commented on her spunky blond haircut, surprised at how much hair she'd grown since her chemotherapy. He was even more surprised when she pulled it straight off her head. Her mom, a hairdresser who was always along for Rebekah's appointments, had a way with wigs. Rebekah had a great attitude and was recovering from advanced metastatic breast cancer. Cindy, still feeling healthy, felt even better after seeing Rebekah.

But if cancer doesn't make a person feel sick, chemotherapy will. Cindy's lymphectomy showed a node with cancerous cells, so her treatment was set at the more aggressive eight sessions, one every three weeks for nearly six months.

One day at the end of January, she and Kevin were shown to a treatment bay off a long room lined with treatment bays, separated by walls with curtains at the front. Cindy waited in the big blue treatment chair while Kevin sat and stood, stood and sat. Patients watched small TVs that floated on long adjustable arms in each bay, and Cindy and Kevin turned theirs on and flipped channels. A nurse came and set up an intravenous anti-nausea drip, then returned every half hour to start three IV bags of colorless Cytoxan, one after another.

Midway, another nurse arrived with two enormous syringes of Adriamycin. She put on thick, opaque blue gloves and injected the bright red poison slowly through a port in the middle of the IV line. Cindy chewed ice chips. This drove blood from the fast-reproducing cells in her mouth, temporarily slowing cell division and preventing mouth sores.

Cindy retched violently all that night and most of the next day. The following day, she went out and ordered a wig.

She dreaded losing the curls Kevin had helped her learn to cherish. From time to time over the years, he'd asked her never to cut her hair. She worried that her baldness, on top of all the other difficulties that her treatment would cause the family, would be a real test of their marriage.

Also, she and her college friend Stephanie had a decade-old ritual of driving a couple of hours to Pittsburgh every two months to shop and have their hair done. They'd been going to the same stylist, Valerie, for eight or nine of those years. More recently, they'd gotten into the habit of having a margarita with lunch at Chi-Chi's afterward. The trips had become more special for them since Cindy had stopped working in Morgantown. She would miss the ritual.

Cindy got the call a few days later that her wig had arrived and, on a cold, sunny Monday in February, she headed to the Clarksburg Beauty Academy after work to have it fitted. Kevin went along, and so did Monica, Dr. Douglas's office assistant and Cindy's coworker and friend.

On the main floor of the beauty school, cutting stations stretched back in two parallel rows under chandeliers, now dark. The high room echoed and glowed, lit from offices on a windowed balcony. Cindy, Kevin, and Monica headed up steps toward the lights. Cindy poked her head into an office.

"Hello, Babycakes!" she greeted a man she barely knew. She'd met Stephen at an American Cancer Society "Look Good, Feel Better" session, where he volunteered by teaching women how to use makeup and wigs to get through chemotherapy. He'd helped Cindy choose her wig. A tall, effusive person who responded well to such affection, Stephen breezed by with a greeting and showed them into a private office.

A dark-paneled room with an orange carpet, frilly upholstery, dolls, and stuffed animals, "Angie's office" contained a small conference table where Cindy and Monica settled into unmatched chairs. Kevin stood, arms crossed. Soon, Stephen returned to deposit an armload of hair paraphernalia on the table. With a flourish, he pulled the wig out of a surprisingly small box.

"Real hair is very heavy," Stephen told them. Not this wig! Kevin and Monica hefted it while Stephen pinned Cindy's still-full head of hair up in tight twists. Cindy chattered, nervous.

Kevin and Monica watched as Stephen stretched the wig over the spirals of hair on Cindy's head. It was more coppery than Cindy's hair, flouncy, shiny. Stephen explained that many women wear their wigs too low on their foreheads because they're afraid they'll fall off. That, more than anything, he told them, is what makes a wig look fake. He showed Cindy how to wear the wig properly. Then he fluffed it and thinned it in snips with scissors that had teeth like a comb. Cindy looked up expectantly: Kevin sighed and smiled. Monica, known for her inability to lie, smiled too.

Cindy already knew that day at the salon that her hair was about to fall out. A 29-year-old Spine Center patient had told her that his head had itched after chemotherapy, and then he'd lost his hair. Stephen predicted she wouldn't lose all her hair because it was very thick, but her head already itched. On Thursday, just three days later, she noticed tufts of her hair lying on the floor in rooms she walked through.

"Here it comes," she thought.

It came in clumps. She tried to ignore it, but by Saturday she had two big bald spots. She asked Kevin to shave her head. In their kitchen, he and the boys cut her hair with scissors until it was shorter than it had been since she and Kevin had been together. Cindy cried. Elijah consoled her, saying, "Don't cry, Mommy. You have your hair in a box!" She cried some more while Kevin shaved her bald with his mom and dad's electric clippers.

When they were done, he said, "Okay, cut mine."

Surprised and appreciative, she shaved his head, too.

———

Now, bald, Cindy felt sick. As if to underscore it, when Rebekah, the breast cancer patient, returned Monday for routine tests, she didn't look right. She was puffy, white. Rebekah hadn't been feeling right either; she'd been lightheaded, and sometimes dizzy. The magnetic resonance imaging (MRI) test confirmed it: a new lesion on her brain. Dr. Douglas wanted to observe the lesion for a month. Cindy felt worried for their patient. She felt worried for herself.

She wore the wig to her second chemotherapy session. It looked fancier than her usual style, but natural enough. Dr. Abraham knew Cindy had gotten sick after the first session three weeks earlier: Kevin had called wanting something to stop the vomiting. It had broken Cindy's heart for Elijah to see her throwing up, then just sitting on a stool by the toilet waiting to throw up again. Abraham had called every day for a week after that.

"Are you trying to kill me?" she'd asked him in frustration once on the phone.

"Well," he'd said, "that is sort of the idea—but then we pull you back, just in time." That had made her laugh.

In the office, Abraham told her that her nausea was extreme. Although he still thought it best for her to continue working, he was concerned that her work with other cancer patients was making her anxious and contributing to her chemotherapy sickness. They would try a different combination of anti-nausea medications this time. When he reminded her that she would need eight treatments, not six as she'd remembered, she glared and joked, "You can go now!"

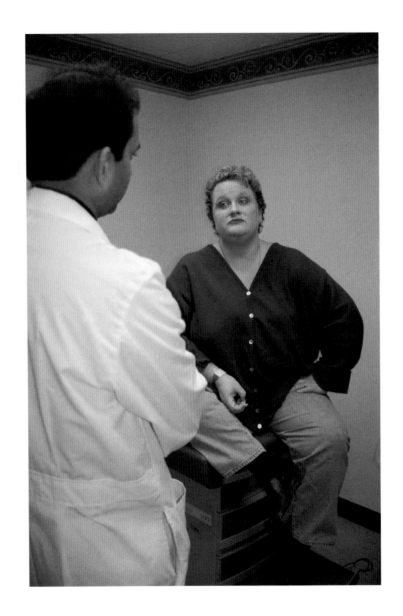

"As a nurse, I have the control and direction over my patient's care," Cindy reflects. "Now, all of a sudden, I was the patient and all these other people were telling me what I had to do to survive."

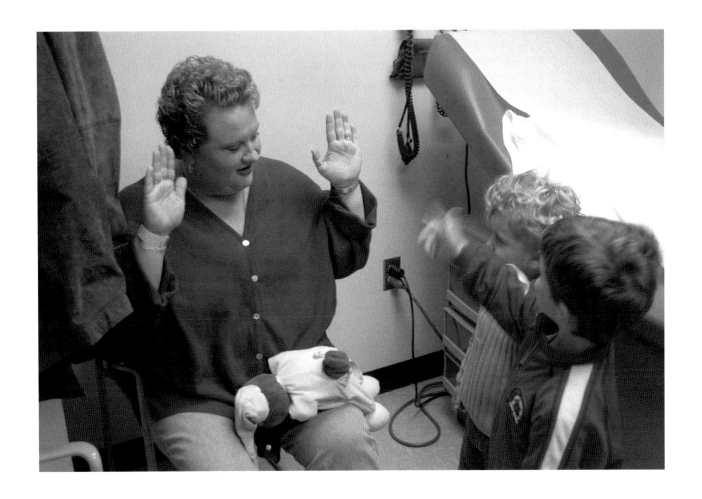

Elijah and Noah play with their mom while waiting for Dr. Abraham at the Mary Babb Randolph Cancer Center in Morgantown. However, the boys weren't present at every appointment. "They always wanted to go, but I never wanted them to see me get chemo," says Cindy.

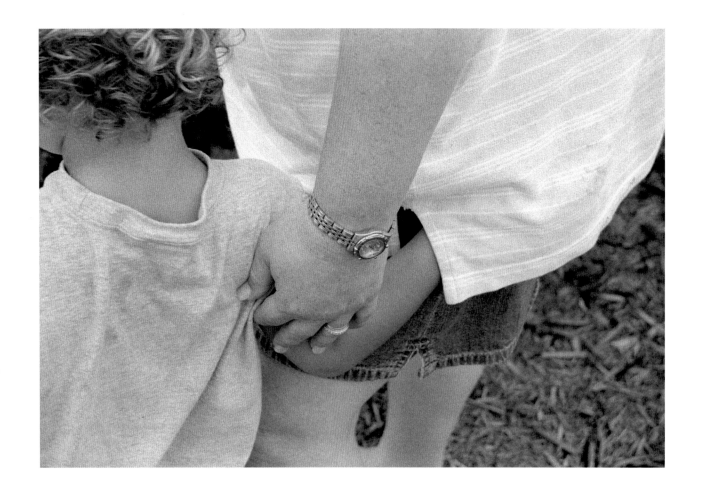

One thing Cindy tried to keep as normal as possible during her treatment was her relationship with sons Elijah and Noah. "Elijah would get so emotional. He was more protective," Cindy said.

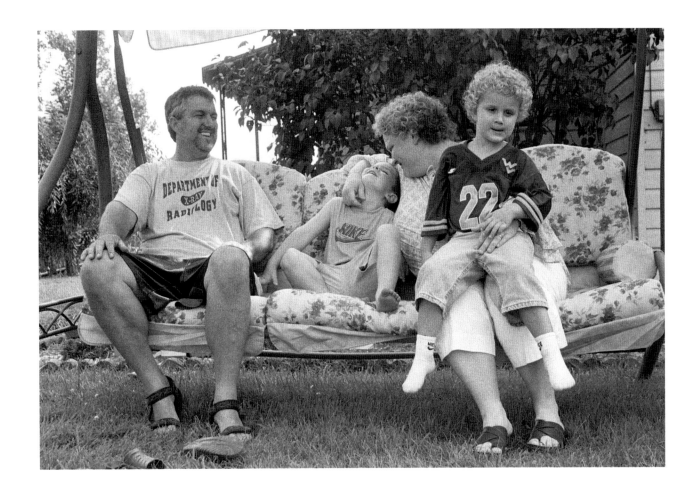

Kevin, Cindy, Elijah, and Noah relax outside on their swing. "I think it was difficult for the kids to understand that I needed to rest, or that Daddy's reading the books instead of me," Cindy says of the boys' reactions to her illness.

Then the second treatment. Kevin sat with her, as he did through every session. When the nurse arrived, Cindy sang out, "There she is, with my toxins!" Mainly, chemotherapy meant a couple of hours of daytime TV. They watched the winter Olympics and "Days of Our Lives." At the end Cindy was drowsy, and Kevin drove her home.

This time, Cindy didn't get so sick. She established a routine of taking every third Thursday and Friday off work: Thursdays for treatments, with Fridays and weekends to recover. She was back at work each Monday and made the time up in the weeks before the next treatment came around. Dr. Douglas openly admired Cindy's strength. He held her up as an inspiration for his back patients: "What are you complaining about? She had chemotherapy last week."

At home and around the office Cindy covered her head with just a bandana, which she called a "do-rag." But she wore the wig in public, especially with patients. Dr. Douglas disliked the wig. He preferred her natural look, even bald, to any pretense. Whenever she put the wig on before seeing patients, he would ask her, "What do you want to put that thing on for?" But she didn't want the patients to know she was sick, didn't want sympathy, didn't want to scare them.

One day in the OR, though, wearing a bandana, she ran into Dr. Kennedy. She never wore the wig in surgery because it was hot and itchy, and it distracted her. Dr. Kennedy told her he thought that not many women could pull off a bald head, but she was one of them. She started to wonder if it might be all right to see patients without the wig. Dr. Douglas was telling all their patients about her cancer anyway. And, really, the wig was about as uncomfortable as being bald. She took a chance without it one day and found that the patients didn't mind at all. So few patients even noticed her baldness that she was unable later to recall her first day in clinic without the wig.

And so her treatment continued through the winter. Another AC session in March. Meanwhile, Rebekah's lesion grew under observation, and they referred her for specialized surgery in Pittsburgh. Another AC in April. The following week, the Spine Center lost four patients to cancer.

Cancer within and all around her, Cindy took her first Taxol treatment on a humid morning in May. Sparse, fine hairs wafted over her scalp when she would let anyone peek under her bandana. Taxol, at least, would not make her nauseous—just sore for a few days.

She still moved stiffly when Rebekah returned. Things were bad with her. Not only had the Pittsburgh surgery failed to stop the tumor, but a head wound from the earlier surgery would not heal, and needed to be closed again. They referred Rebekah to Dr. Kennedy for that. Worse still, Rebekah had yet another lesion, this one on her lung. She underwent new rounds of chemotherapy and radiation and looked paler and more swollen than ever.

Rebekah pushed Cindy's edge as a nurse. Her sickness just hit too close to home. After Cindy's second Taxol treatment, another visit from Rebekah. Her head wound remained: Dr. Kennedy had decided she wouldn't live through the surgery. Her skin was dusky, and she moved slowly. A third Taxol. Another visit from Rebekah. All of Cindy's training and ideals told her to be compassionate, but she couldn't help thinking she was seeing herself in five years. She wanted to run.

Some evenings, after hours, Cindy and Dr. Douglas talked about patients, about family, and about cancer. Though she never let him think it was too hard for her to work, she sometimes confessed her deep tiredness. Dr. Douglas, who dipped snuff, said, "They've found your cancer, they just haven't found mine yet." He'd already escaped death once, and if he ever had cancer, he told her, he would just go to a beach somewhere. Maybe he would, maybe not, she thought, but cancer wasn't going to take over her life. He'd see.

—·—

Finally, the last chemotherapy session came on a hot, hot day in July. Cindy and Kevin arrived anxious. She'd slept poorly. Dr. Abraham hugged her and shook her hand. He shook Kevin's hand, then stood gazing at Cindy with arms crossed, smiling.

Dr. Abraham was happy. Cindy wasn't. She dreaded life after chemotherapy. Every bump she'd find now, she'd think it was cancer. She took her Taxol quietly, under a blanket, watching "Days of Our Lives." No sign of triumph crossed her face as her last bag of toxins emptied. She didn't feel done. She didn't think she'd ever feel done.

———

Cindy and Kevin took the kids to Cincinnati, to Kings Island amusement park. She had kept working all the way through chemotherapy, and was only 20 hours behind after eight months of the ordeal. After a month's break, the only treatment left was six weeks of radiation, a few minutes every weekday. As the time after her last chemotherapy session lengthened, she began to feel certain that she would finish without taking sick leave.

But then, in mid-August, before Cindy's break was over, Rebekah's mom called. She told Cindy that Rebekah had passed out by the pool and was admitted through the ER.

Cindy thought it was probably the end for Rebekah. Dr. Douglas insisted that she go with him to visit her—"made" her go, she felt, though her own conscience told her she should do it.

Rebekah lay on the bed, gray, drooling. She was extremely weak. Cindy sat on the edge of her bed and talked with her about everyday things. Rebekah wasn't making much sense. When Cindy left the room she cried and cried. It had happened so fast. She was scared. She wanted to see her sons grow up.

On September 16, 2002, Rebekah died. Her mom called Cindy to tell her about the arrangements. Although she sometimes attended patients' funerals, Cindy couldn't make herself go to this one. She and Dr. Douglas sent a big bouquet of flowers.

———

Cindy was halfway through six weeks of radiation treatments when Rebekah died. It was hard to put it out of her mind. Rebekah had looked so healthy not all that long ago. She'd had such a good attitude! And excellent care. How could this have happened? Cindy felt physically and emotionally exhausted. She needed a break.

But what she wanted still more was to work until the end of her treatment. She forced herself to get through those last weeks of daily appointments and to do her job cheerfully each day. A few days before her final radiation treatment, she started warning Dr. Douglas to clean off his desk, because she was going to dance on it.

On October 10, Cindy returned from radiation for the last time. Dr. Douglas sat working at his desk. It was as cluttered as usual.

"I told you so," she said, deciding to satisfy herself with that.

Dr. Douglas smiled a strange smile, a smile that made Cindy wonder. Had he set her up from the beginning?

She asked for a *real* day off.

———

Cindy's hair grew in dark brown with gray, curlier than before, a little wiry. Her uncle thought he recognized her dad's trademark Afro. Trying to blow it straighter only made it frizzy.

Cindy and Stephanie drove to Pittsburgh in a January snowstorm. Cindy was eager to do something with her hair, though she wasn't sure what. When it was a little shorter, she'd spiked it with gel, and her kids had thought she was cool. Now, though, it was too long for that, and she didn't want to go back to less hair.

Valerie, all dressed in black and holding a huge takeout cup from a coffee shop, met Cindy and Stephanie by the coat rack in a trendy downtown salon. "You guys drive so far, but you're never late," she said, "no matter how snowy it is!" She hugged Cindy. Much had happened since they'd last seen each other. She gave them smocks and took them upstairs to her station.

Valerie had only known Cindy with long hair, so she was excited to try something new. While Valerie, hands in bright green gloves, brushed color onto Stephanie's hair, Cindy looked through a style book, pointing out colors and cuts she liked. They chose a color more like her natural red: "Blazing Brown" mixed with "Sandy Gold." Stephanie's hair soaked up dye while Valerie brushed a highlighter onto random tips of Cindy's hair. She folded them into foil packets, then brushed the color they'd chosen onto the remaining hair.

They had a lot to talk about. Valerie had had a daughter since she'd last seen Cindy, and they shared kid photos. Cindy talked about her treatment. She told Valerie that Kevin had held her hair back when she puked—when she had hair—and that he never missed an appointment. She wouldn't be considered "cancer-free," she explained, until she was without cancer for five years.

And Valerie told her she'd had her own cancer scare just two months earlier. She'd barely been able to think during the day it had taken to find out if it was malignant. She'd spilled hair color all over a wall at work, and wrecked her car. The false alarm gave her more sympathy for what Cindy had gone through.

"I was surprised to learn that it's more aggressive in young people. I mean, that's not what you'd think," Valerie said.

Cindy said nothing.

Dark streaks stained the sink as Valerie rinsed the dye from Cindy's hair. The gold highlights stood out from the brown. It felt good to have hair and to lie back and have it washed. Cindy closed her eyes and inhaled the oatmeal and honey aroma of Valerie's latest favorite shampoo. She smiled.

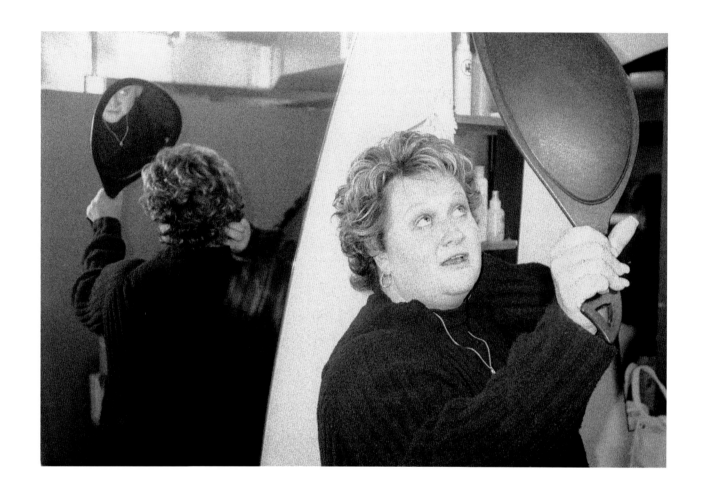

During a visit to her stylist in Pittsburgh, Cindy checks her regrown hair.

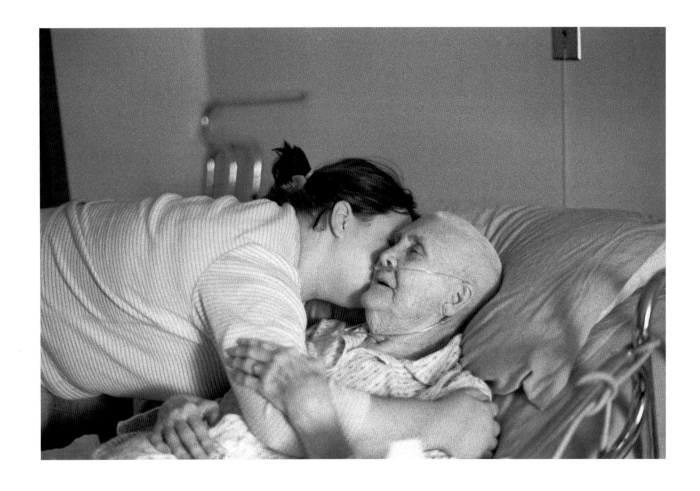

After more than a year of working on the story of Geraldine Thomas' struggle with lung cancer, student Sally Ann Cruikshank and Geraldine share final good byes. Geraldine died a few days later. "It's been really hard," Sally Ann admits. "I lost my mother to cancer. It's one of the reasons why I wanted to do this project. I thought about how I would like to have something like this to look at." Photo by Barbara Griffin

Listening for Cancer Stories

by DAVID G. ALLEN

In late June 2000, I proposed the cancer project to David C. Hardesty, Jr., president of West Virginia University. A week later, the project had the green light. My idea was that there was much to be learned from listening in detail to the stories of everyday people battling cancer.

At the time, I was very concerned about protecting patient privacy. While I knew that many cancer patients would willingly talk about their ordeals, I did not know if they would submit to a public reading. That so many patients were willing to share their lives with us is a gesture that we hold dear to our hearts.

The men and women you meet in *Cancer Stories* are the bravest of the brave; they personify courage and integrity better than any model that I know. Please cherish the moments that you spend with them; for they, and their families, have made great personal sacrifices to bring you their stories.

When the faculty of the Perley Isaac Reed School of Journalism and the medical staff of the Mary Babb Randolph Cancer Center began to define this project's parameters, there was agreement that *Cancer Stories* could be a wonderful publication if properly done. This was the turning point, and the project took on new dimensions. No longer would this be an academic exercise for doctors in training. If anything, the feeling of the medical staff was that these stories would greatly benefit the public, both as an educational tool and as an emotional comfort.

215

As you undoubtedly know, saying it and doing it are usually a continent apart. And most of the time, academic buildings on the same university campus are poles, if not planets, apart. That our young reporters blended into the fabric of this tapestry so completely as to be unnoticed, and yet captured the realism of each day in the life of a cancer patient, is a testament to this university, its faculty and staff, and its students.

The Journalism School and the Cancer Center formulated a plan so comprehensive that success was all but guaranteed from the outset. For example, the journalism students began their assignments by attending classes oncologists taught. Thus, they had the medical knowledge and background to report their stories intelligently. These same students also attended classes in immersion journalism, which taught them precisely how to pursue the in-depth stories they had been assigned.

Of this plan and the efforts by the faculty and medical staff, I offer my praise. The preparation to undertake this project was well thought out, and the execution perfect.

As for proposing the idea for this project, I think that I just happened to be the stew pot with the right bones. Consider the following:

I graduated from the Virginia Military Institute with a Bachelor of Arts in economics. VMI did not offer journalism courses. However, I worked on the "Cadet" newspaper staff for three years. While primarily a photographer and photo editor, I also did about every other job available, including selling ads. This experience allowed me to know just how energetic and accomplished college students can be when it comes to journalistic pursuits.

Both of my parents died from cancer. I remember well the ordeals with which my family dealt.

In spring 2000, I was asked to serve on the advisory board of the Cancer Center. Knowing the staff of the Cancer Center as well as so many on staff at WVU Hospitals gave me the insight that these professionals possessed the compassion and caring to nurture *Cancer Stories*.

And finally, I was left paralyzed after a car accident in 1994. For the next five months, I lived in hospitals. I knew firsthand how patients react to life-changing injuries and illnesses. It was during my four-month physical rehabilitation stay at Craig Hospital in Denver where I learned that talking about one's personal crisis can often be as therapeutic as medical treatment.

I ask you: How could I not propose this project?

———

When we began this venture, I had but one demand: I wanted true reporting. My exact comment was, "I don't want *Chicken Soup*!" However, it was not my intention to demean this popular series of inspirational articles. *Chicken Soup*, to use the pun, is heartening. But to gloss over the torment of a cancer diagnosis or to speak only of the survivors could never support the goals of this project. To this end, the Perley Isaac Reed School of Journalism students were faithful and unbiased reporters, and they have delivered a remarkable and honest catalog of the facets of life—as well as the range of emotions—that we call the human spirit.

When I was a teenager, my cousin, Margaret Thrasher, died from cancer. She was 14. Back then, cancer was barely treatable. Her death came just a decade after the oral polio vaccine was invented. At once, it was an era of so much hope and promise, yet still a dark age filled with dragons in the shadows, cancer being the worst of them.

My mother's cancer began with skin tumors and then spread internally. She was 75 when diagnosed. Her life had been extended nearly 20 years by another medical miracle, the heart pacemaker. For those years with her, our family was very grateful.

James, my father, was diagnosed with lung cancer after having a computerized axial tomography (CAT) scan to determine whether he had injuries from a fall. The scan showed a tumor in one lung, but he felt no symptoms. He was going on 88, and did not undergo any treatment or surgery. For him, his decision was the right one, because he did not want to suffer a stroke or debilitation of any kind. He was sick only for the last few days of his life.

My father was fond of repeating the old adages that his elders passed down to him. He told me this one many years earlier: "Pneumonia is an old man's friend." And in the end, it was true for him.

After *Cancer Stories* got underway, my oldest brother, Jim, died in 2001 from lung and liver cancer. Chemotherapy gave him a year more than the 62 that Nature had planned, and in that brief time, he was able, as they say, to get his affairs in order. Though his prognosis was poor at the outset, watching his tumors shrink on successive scans was a medical miracle, if only a temporary one.

We have come a long way in four decades. By learning even more about cancer, we will continue to make progress in curing it. To this end, I believe that the feedback from patients is just as important and integral a part of the investigation as are the test tubes and imaging machines.

That Lance Armstrong survived cancer with today's medicines is an impressive feat. That Lance Armstrong, cancer survivor, then went on to win another Tour de France shows that our attitudes toward cancer have changed dramatically. No longer are we amenable to just surviving cancer. We now have it in our psyche that we must recapture our quality of life to be completely cured.

⩔